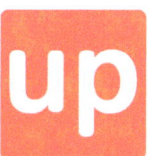

Improve Reading Comprehension

for ages 6-12

Elena K. Andreou - Special educator, BSc, MA, MEd

Upbility Publications LTD | 81–83 Grivas Digenis Avenue, Nicosia, 1090 Cyprus

E-mail: info@upbility.eu

www.upbility.net

SKU: EN-EB1138

Author: Elena K. Andreou - Special educator, BSc, MA, MEd

Pagination/Illustration: Zanna Katsafana

Improve Reading Comprehension
for ages 6-12

TABLE OF CONTENTS

THEORETICAL PART

1. READING COMPREHENSION DEVELOPMENT PHASES

Acquiring reading comprehension skills is vital for the children's school success and cognitive development. For teachers and parents, one thing they must always have in mind is that reading comprehension takes time to develop. As a matter of fact, it evolves through five different phases and keeps improving in someone's adult years.

These five phases are:

1) **Pre-reading phase**
2) **Initial reading phase**
3) **Practice phase**
4) **Extensive reading phase**
5) **Comprehension phase**

1.1. Pre-reading phase

The pre-reading phase is the period before children learn the mechanics of reading, mainly the pre-school years. During that time, children acquire these five fundamental sets of skills necessary for learning to read and comprehend written speech:

1) Basic visual perception skills: Visual perception skills such as visual closure, visual figure-ground discrimination, visual form constancy, visual memory, visual discrimination, and visual-spatial relations are honed during the pre-reading phase. They all later contribute to the child mastering the reading mechanism and achieving fluency.

2) Phonological awareness: It's the ability to recognize and manipulate the sounds of words and understand that words are made of syllables, and syllables are made of phonemes. The child must learn to use syllables and phonemes appropriately (e.g., join syllables and phonemes to create words, break words into syllables and phonemes, and manipulate or drop existing syllables and phonemes to create new words).

3) Vocabulary development: The child must develop a vocabulary and grasp the semantic meaning of different phrases and words through semantic correlations.

4) Picture-word association: The child must associate pictures with corresponding words or phrases and understand that writing can represent pictures, concepts, or ideas.

5) Understanding the function of writing: In this phase, a child must begin to understand the basic structure and communicative function of writing: we write to send messages and read to receive those messages. Also, the child must familiarize themselves with writing and reading orientation: we read by moving our eyes from top to bottom and from left to right.

Most of these skills are developed through children's daily activities and interaction with adults and other children, as well as through special education programs and activities in early childhood education.

1.2. Initial reading phase

Children begin to make a first letter-sound association—by combining letters with their corresponding sounds—and visually recognize small words. At the same time, they gradually master the reading mechanism by decoding two-syllable or three-syllable words. They also begin to practice reading multi-syllable words. First, they read simple-structured words (CV), and then, they proceed to complex-structured words containing consonant clusters (CCV) and diphthongs. In this phase, children begin to combine the words they read to understand the meaning of a sentence or a small sentence sequence (e.g., a short text). Hence, it's essential for children to be exposed to a variety of simple texts and encouraged to read regularly.

1.3. Practice phase

Children develop and master their reading skills through continuous practice. In this phase, the young reader goes through several stages to acquire adequate reading comprehension skills:

Visually recognizing words: Children begin to automatically recognize words they have encountered frequently.

Increasing reading speed: Children begin to read faster and more fluently while becoming better at text comprehension.

Improving comprehension: While they keep better at word recognition and faster at decoding, children focus more and more on comprehending the information and ideas that texts convey.

Processing complex texts: Children begin to read more complex texts that include indefinite concepts, complex ideas, and subtle messages.

Developing reading comprehension strategies: Children develop strategies for better understanding texts, such as predicting, retrieving, noting, and problem-solving.

In this phase, the key is exposing children to a variety of text types and encouraging continuous practice. Teachers and parents must provide support and guidance and have realistic expectations regarding children's progress according to each child's overall cognitive level.

1.4. Extensive reading phase

Children further improve their various reading-related skills (visual perception, vocabulary, fluency, and comprehension) and begin to use reading as a tool to expand their knowledge:

❯ **Vocabulary expansion:** Children continue to expand their vocabulary by identifying and understanding more difficult or specialized words. To support their progress, they must read books appropriate to their age and not for younger or older children.

❯ **Critical thinking and analysis:** Children begin to deeply analyze texts and think critically about the included topics, characters, ideas, and techniques.

❯ **Improving reading strategies:** Children continue to develop and improve their reading strategies, such as predicting, summarizing, and evaluating.

❯ **Complex comprehension:** Children begin to comprehend multidimensional texts that may have multiple interpretations or complex structures.

The extensive reading phase is crucial for children to further develop their reading skills. It prepares them for the advanced literary analysis and critical thinking required in their later academic and professional life.

1.5. Comprehension phase

It's the most essential phase in a child's reading development. Children have already acquired the basic reading skills to read more independently and focus on understanding and interpreting the text's content. They can analyze, evaluate, and critique information using specific strategies to improve comprehension. In this phase, reading is transformed from a mechanical process to a combination of active understanding and information processing.

2. READING COMPREHENSION LEVELS

Reading comprehension proficiency is divided into the following levels:

❯ **Verbal level:** It's the stage of literal comprehension. The reader understands basic information, such as facts and the text's easily recognizable details.

Interpretive level: The reader interprets and connects indirect information in the text to comprehend its deeper meaning. They analyze characters, themes, and implications and distinguish the text's various similes, idioms, and metaphors.

Critical level: The reader evaluates and critiques the text using critical thinking, related analysis, and connection to external knowledge and experiences.

Creative level: The reader uses the text's information, ideas, and meanings to express their own ideas or sentences. They can also apply or adapt the text's ideas to new contexts.

Once children have mastered all the reading comprehension stages, we must encourage them to interact with texts of all levels to develop an overall understanding of how to read a text.

3. STRATEGIES FOR DEVELOPING READING COMPREHENSION

Teachers and parents can use several strategies to help children develop their reading comprehension skills, such as:

Predictions and questions: Children are asked to predict how a text continues, provide a different ending, retell the story from the point of a specific character, change the main characters' decisions, and add their own characters. They are also encouraged to ask questions and seek answers in the text. It's important for children to find them within the text and be able to point out where they have found each answer.

To early readers and students with learning difficulties, teachers or parents must provide questions with clear answers within the text. To experienced readers without challenges, the questions must be more difficult, so they are encouraged to process the text to extract the answer. Questions requiring critical thinking are essential as they allow children to seek answers by drawing from their own personal experiences.

Visualization: Children are encouraged to create mental images based on the text. That strategy is usually recommended for beginners and readers with learning difficulties. Visualization improves comprehension and enhances children's memory and their ability to recall the temporal sequence of the events in the text.

Connection to prior knowledge: Learning is considered more effective when new information is somehow connected to the reader's previous knowledge, helping them to better comprehend and memorize information. It's recommended for older children who are going through the extensive reading and comprehension phases where they read to expand their knowledge.

Reading aloud, recording, and discussion: Reading aloud helps children listen to the language in the text and process it. Recording helps children listen to their voice, identify weaknesses (especially in decoding and fluency, e.g., punctuation marks), and consolidate the text's parts they didn't understand while reading. Discussion provides the opportunity for deeper content exploration and critical thinking. Reading aloud and recording are aimed primarily at early readers and students with difficulties. Discussion is aimed at children of all ages and levels.

Using graphic charts & organizational diagrams: Children learn to organize the information found in a text in a visually accessible and clear way. Tools like Venn diagrams, idea maps, and brainstorming help children better understand the connections between different elements in the text and analyze its content more deeply. Graphic diagrams can be used from the first elementary school grades up to the last years of high school.

Applying these strategies to reading practice can significantly improve children's reading comprehension and overall language development skills.

PREFACE

This book contains reading comprehension exercises and texts for early and experienced readers. The initial basic exercises are for helping children understand simple sentences and how written language conveys messages, images, or ideas.

They are followed by exercises of increasing difficulty based on texts and open and close-ended questions. They aim to help children develop auditory comprehension, processing, and memory.

Important reminder: Not all texts are suitable for all children! They should be selected according to each child's particular personality, cognitive skills, and interests.

If a text is too difficult or too easy for the child's current level, the exercise cannot achieve any of its objectives.

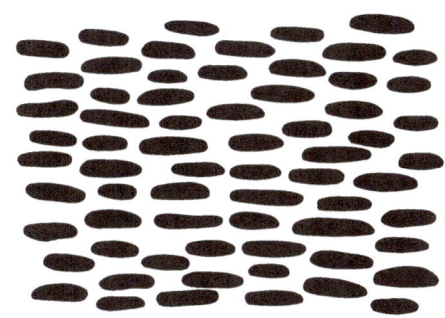

LEVEL 1

Circle the correct answer.

Circle the duck that's in the bag.

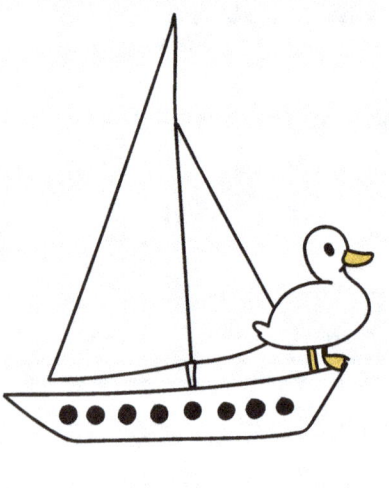
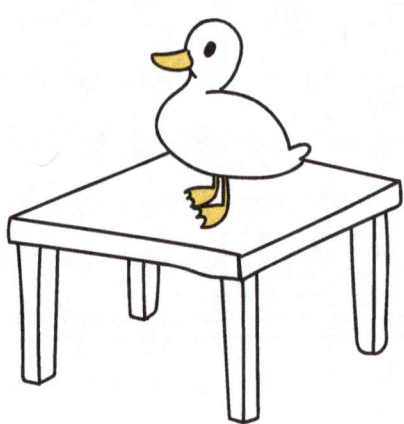
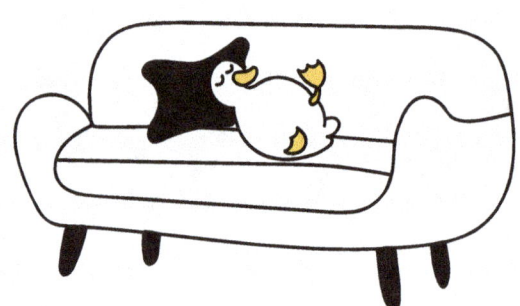
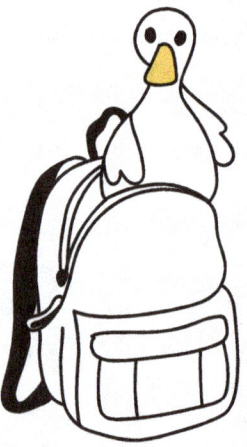
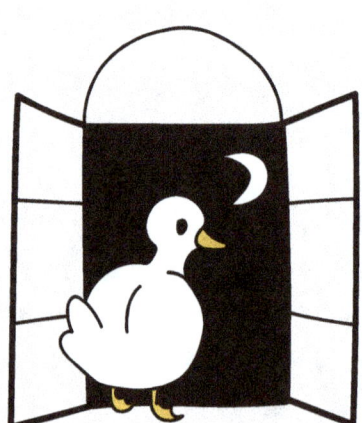

Circle the correct answer.

Circle the brown hat.

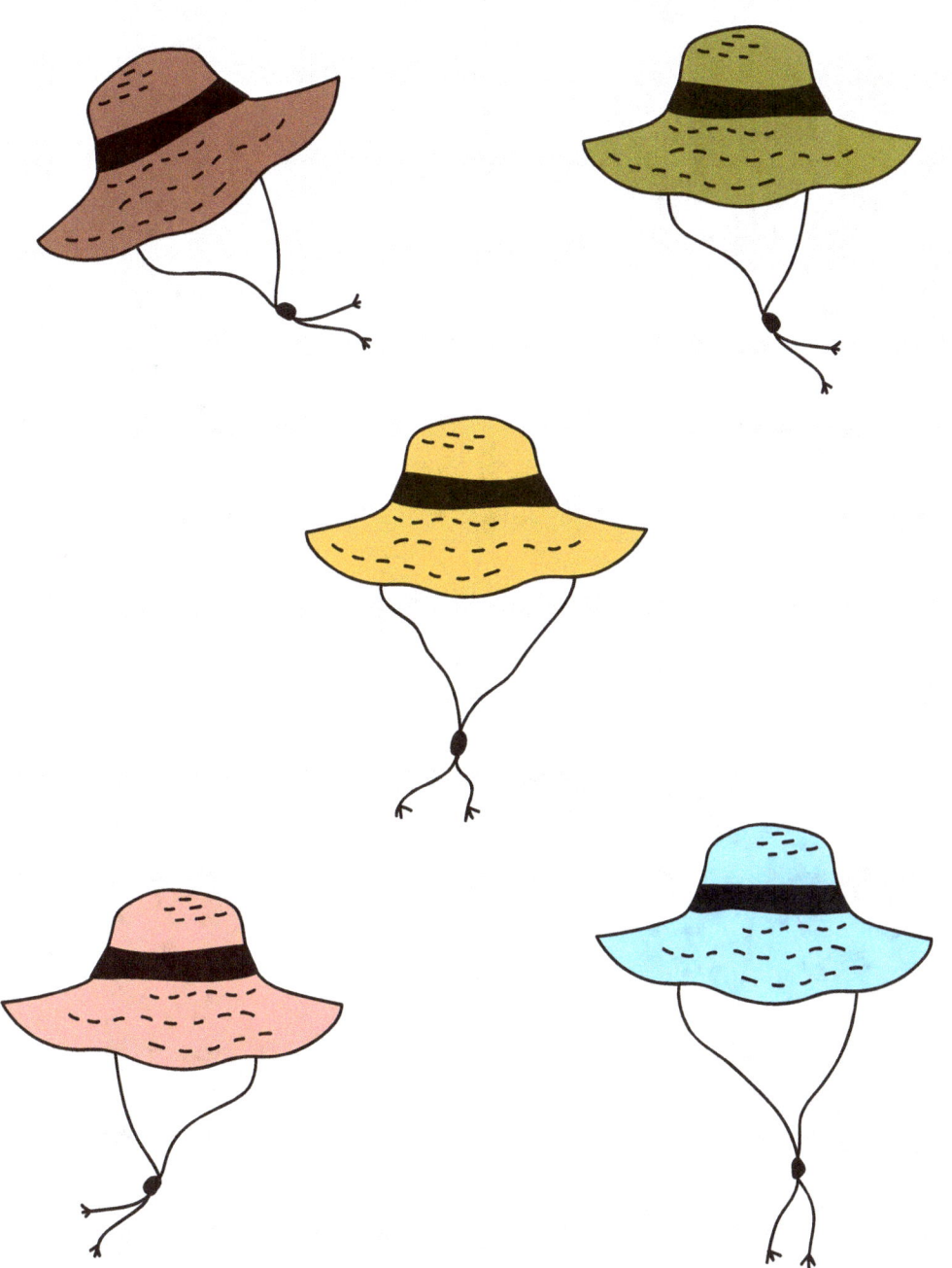

Circle the correct answer.

Circle the vase with the red flowers.

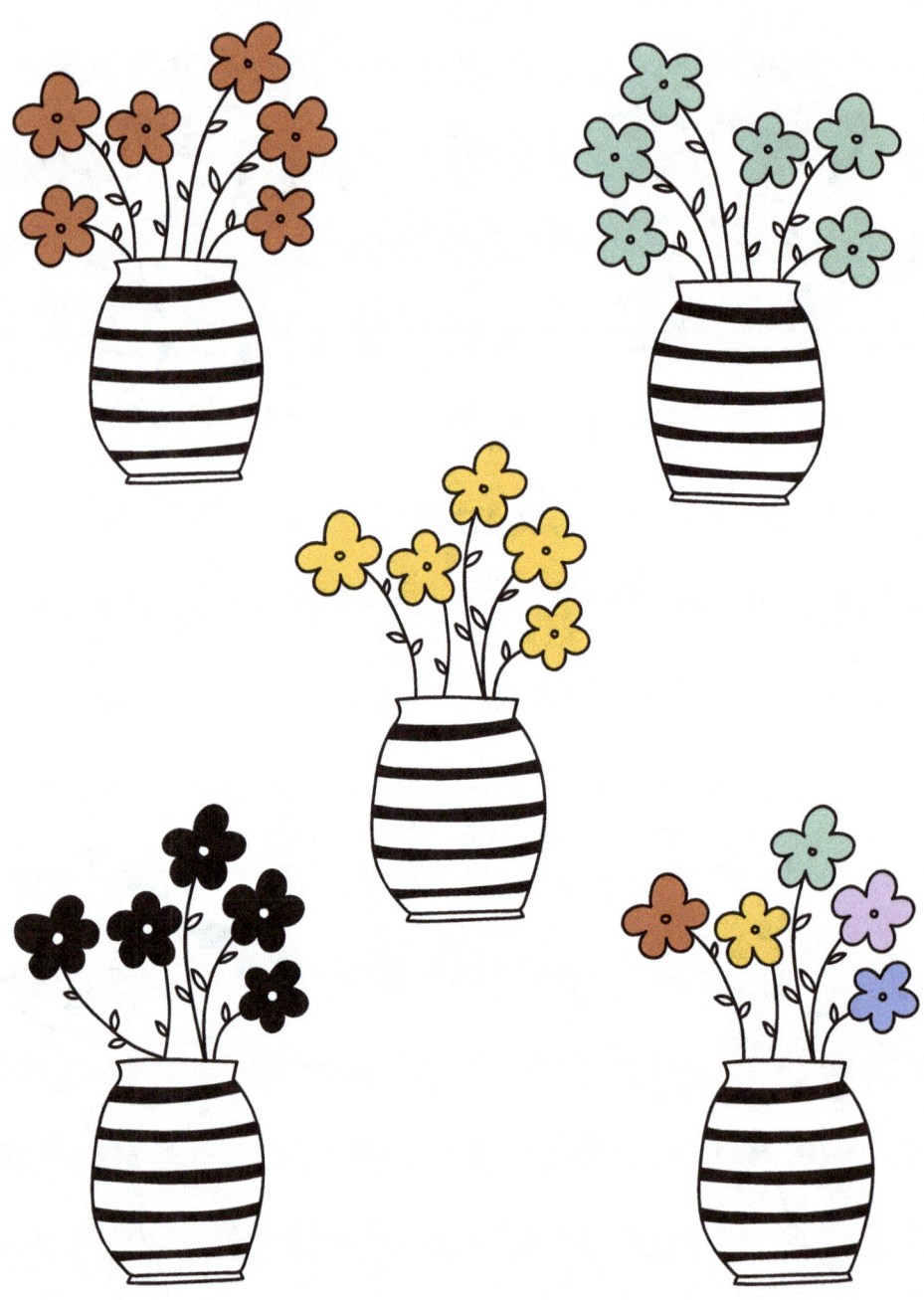

Circle the correct answer.

Circle the blue car.

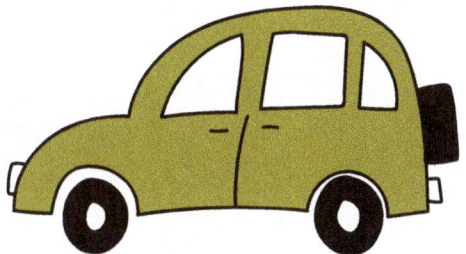
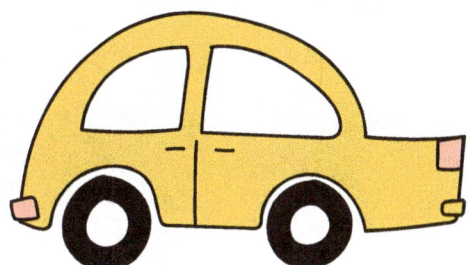

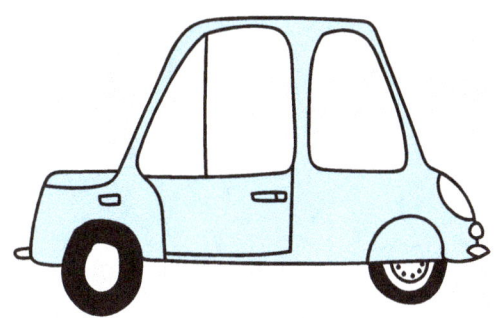

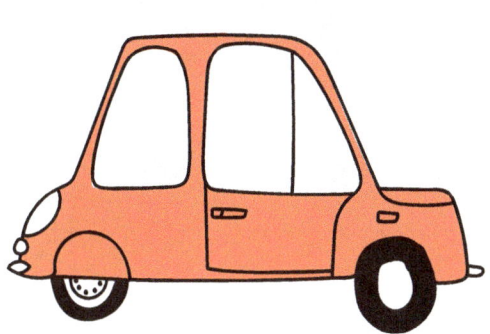
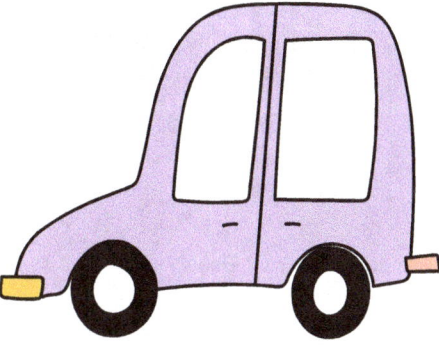

Circle the correct answer.

Circle the last duck.

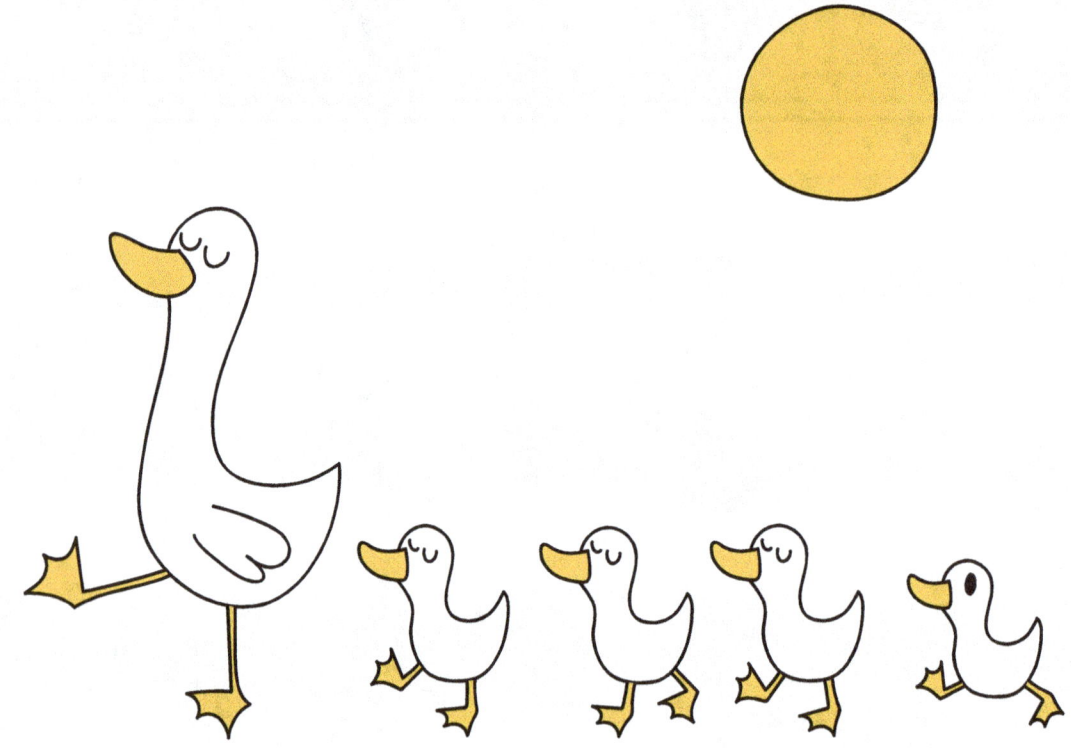

Circle the correct answer.

Circle the boy sitting in the car.

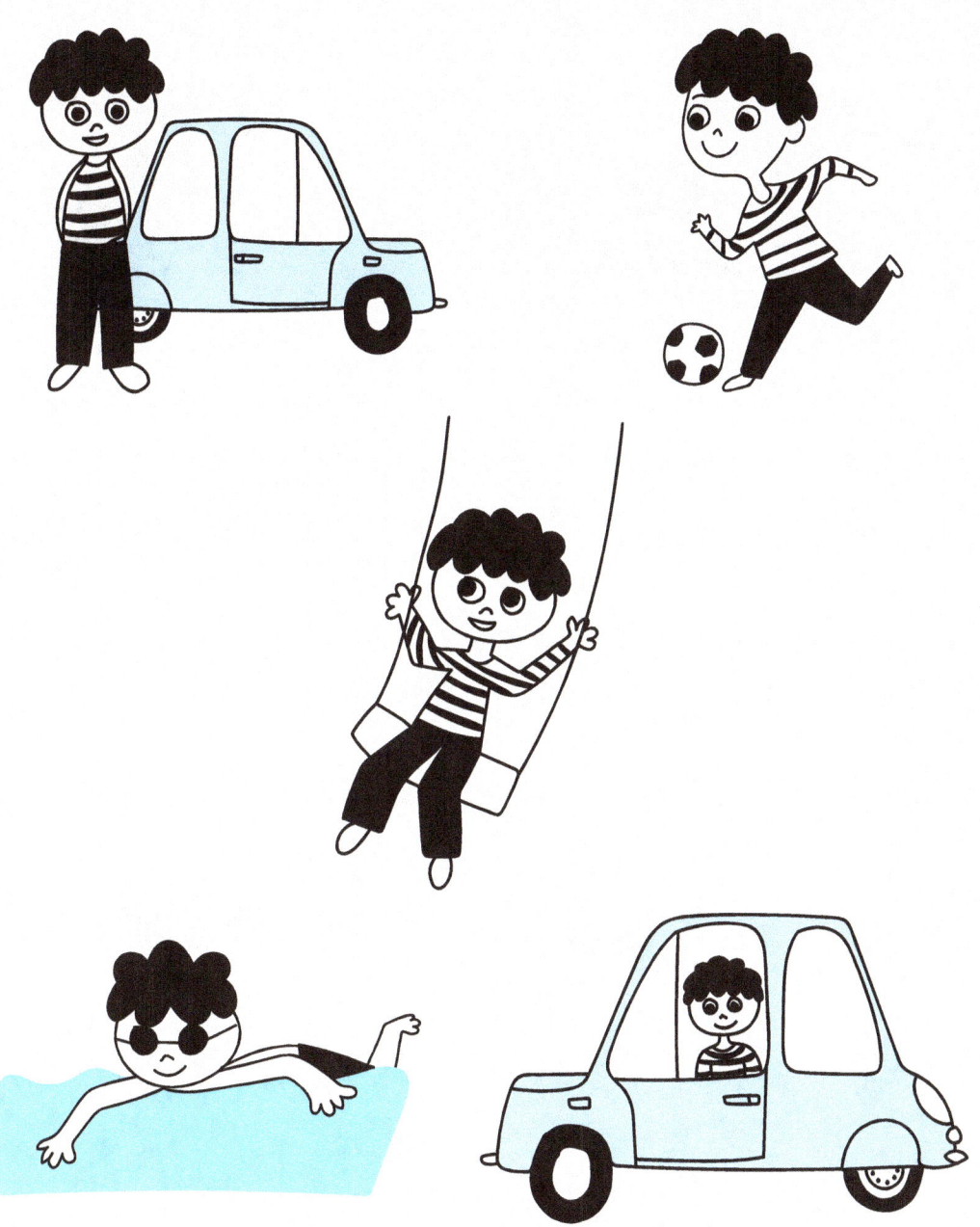

Circle the correct answer.

Circle the dog with the longest tail.

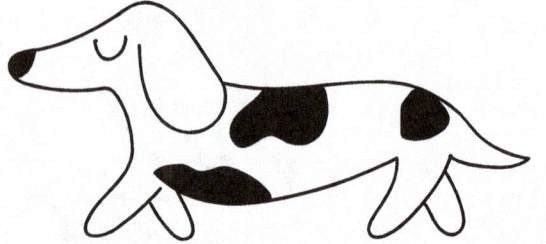
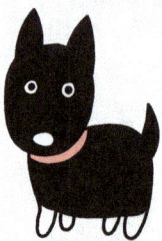
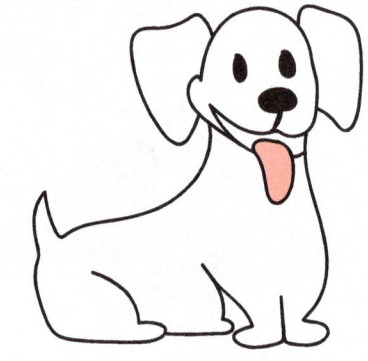
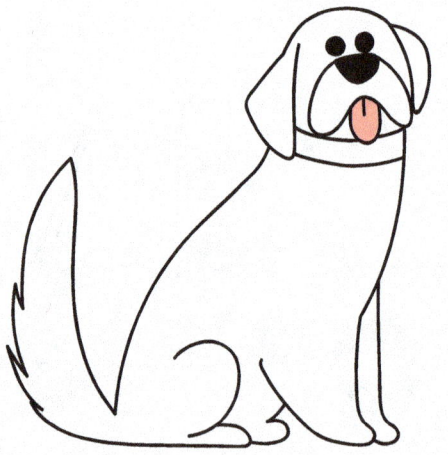
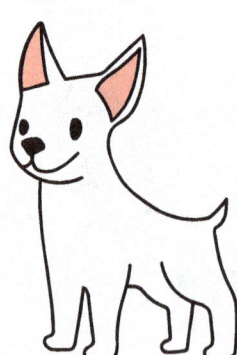

Circle the correct answer.

Circle the tallest boy.

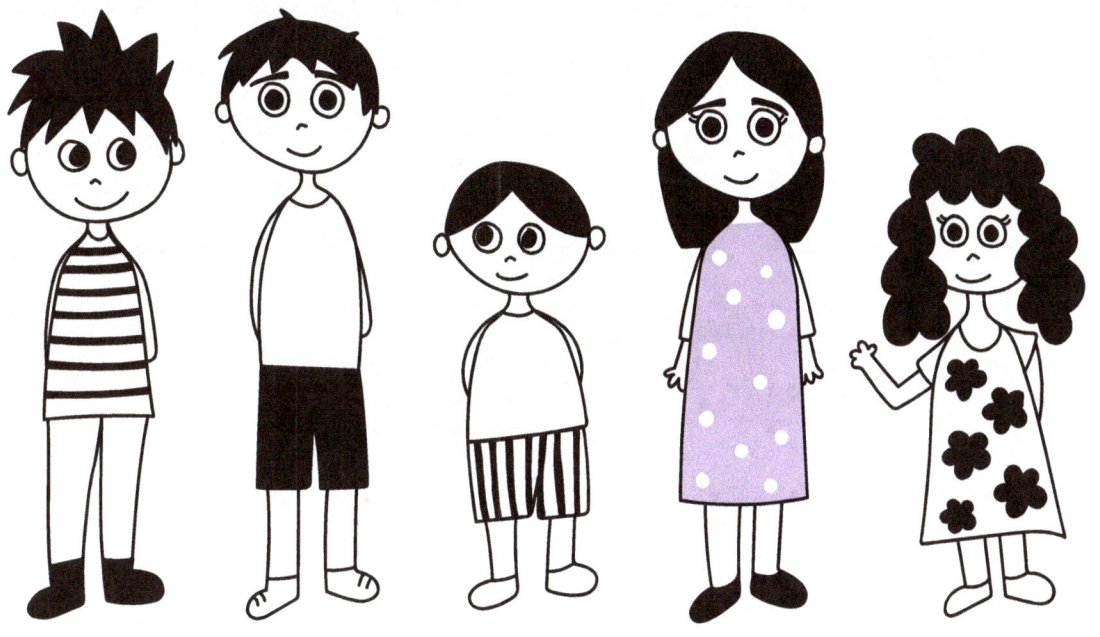

Circle the correct answer.

Circle the orange bike.

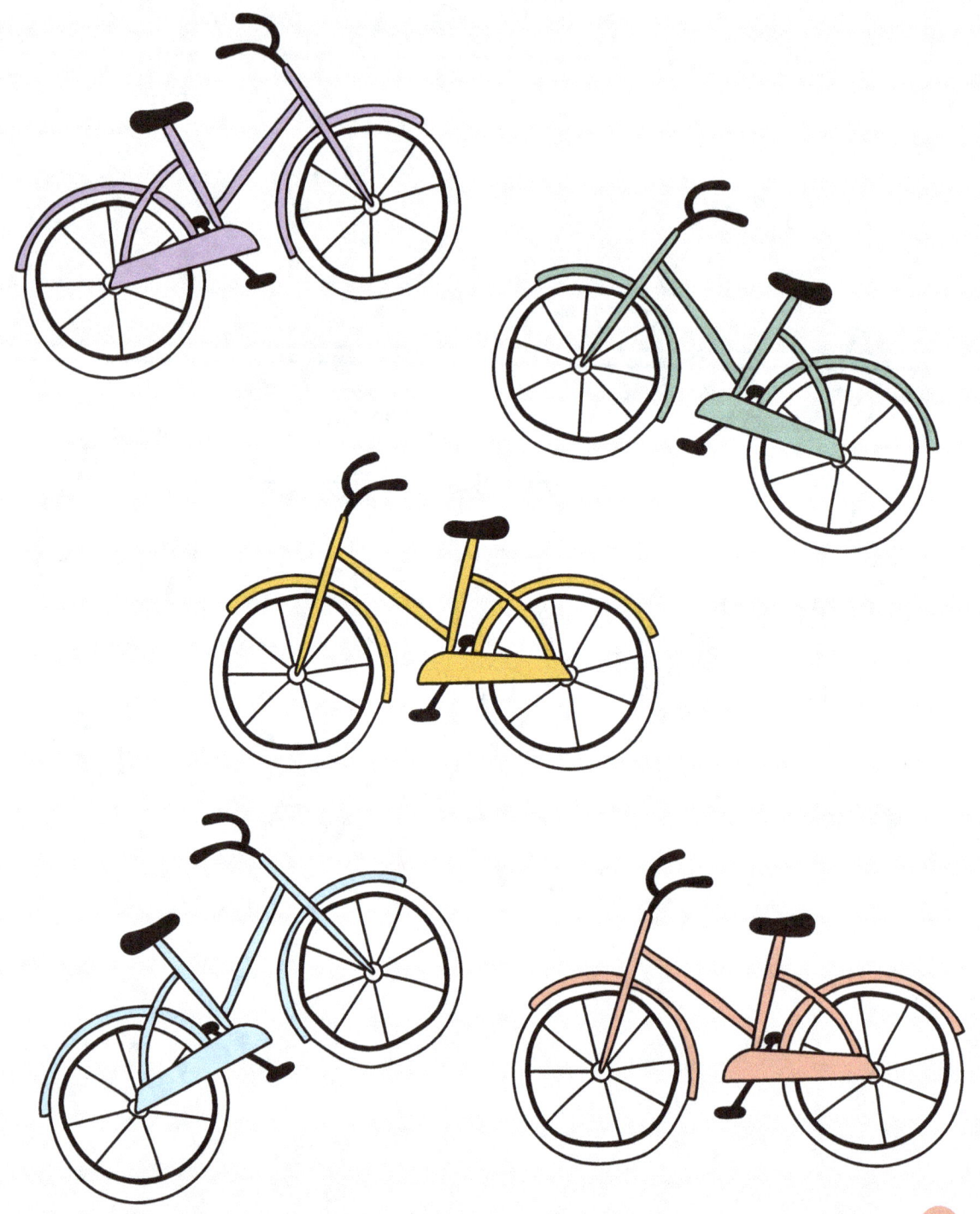

Circle the correct answer.

Circle the kitten wearing a green collar.

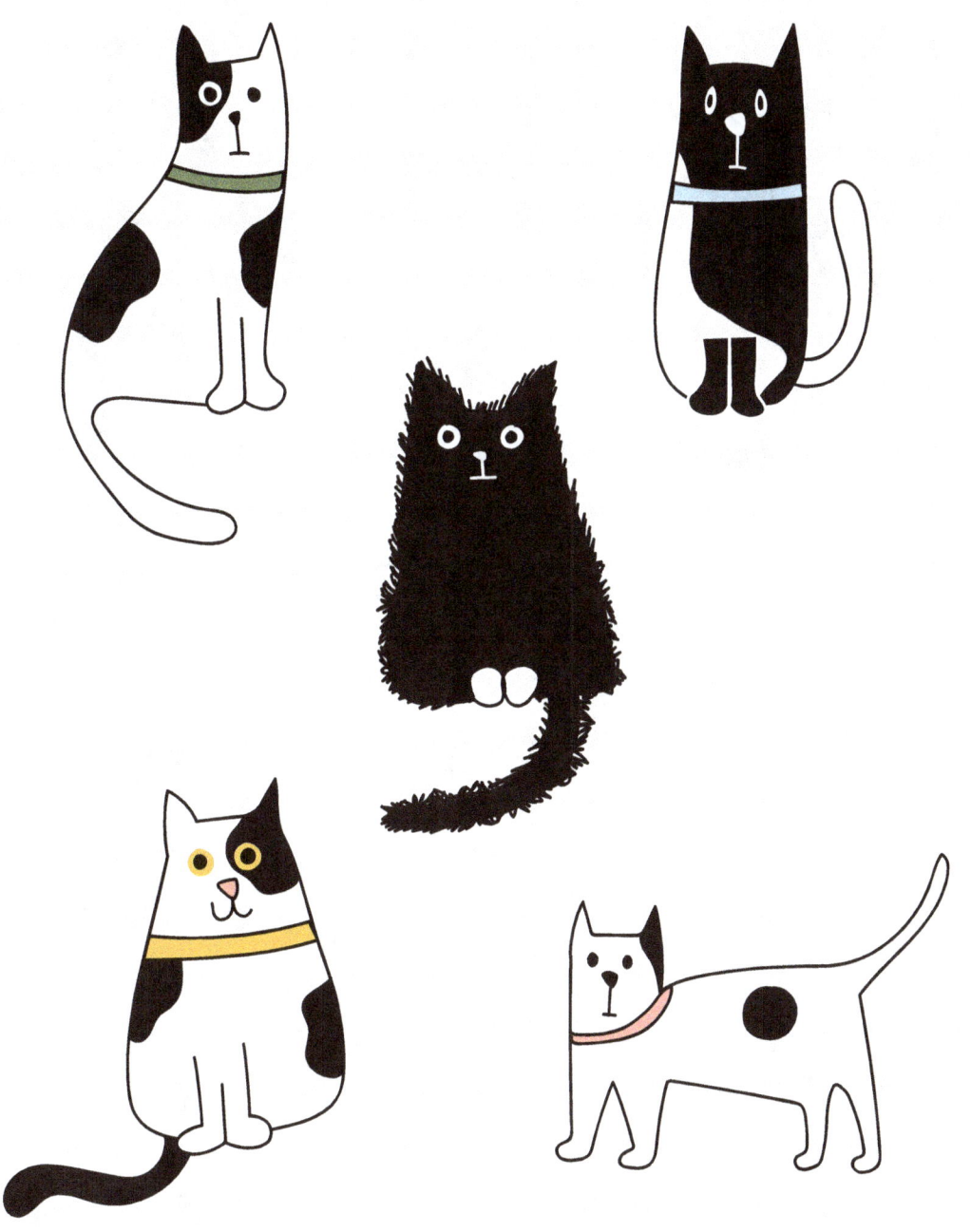

Circle the correct answer.

Circle the girl carrying a yellow bag.

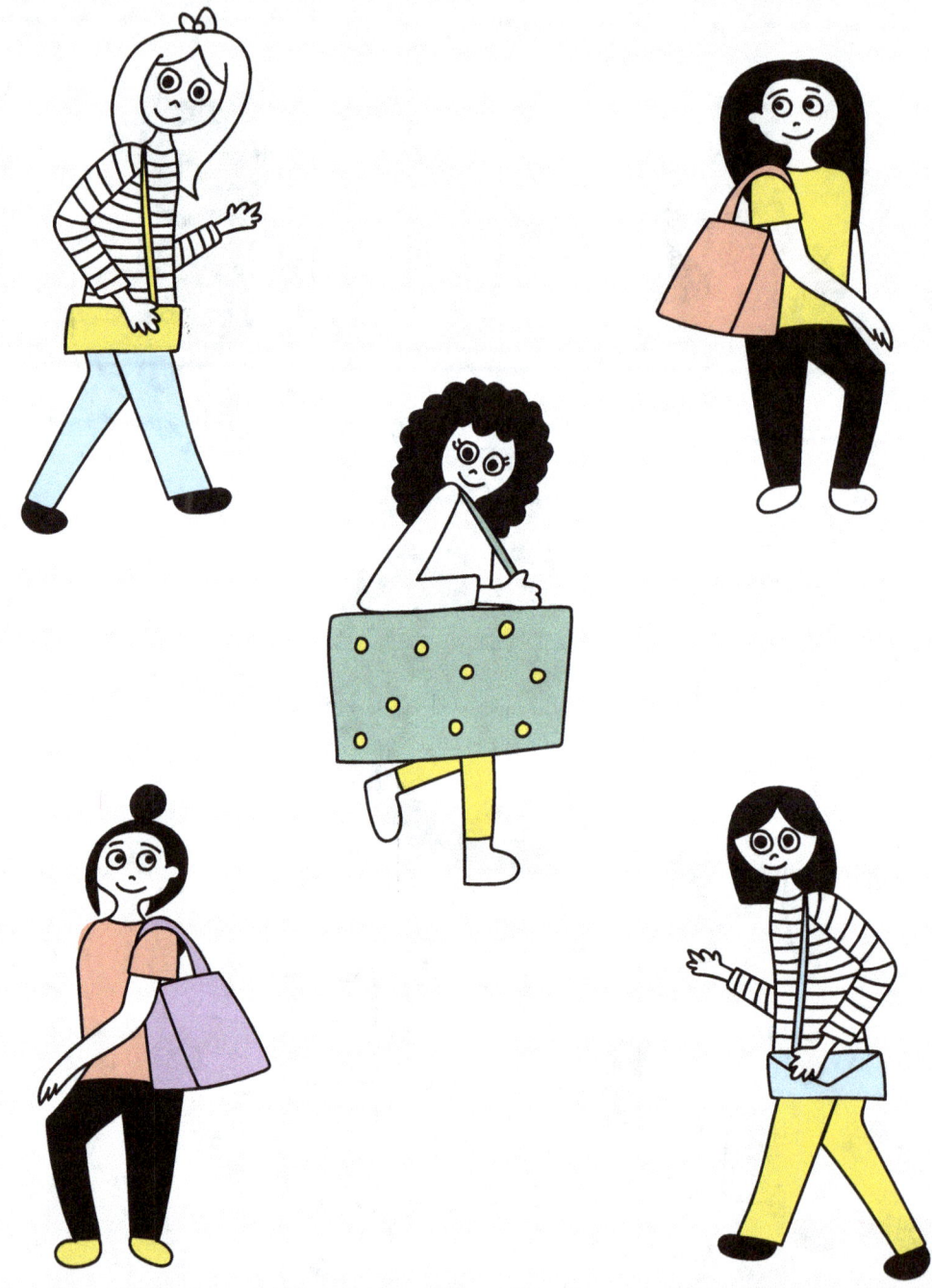

Circle the correct answer.

Circle the pink teddy bear wearing a red t-shirt.

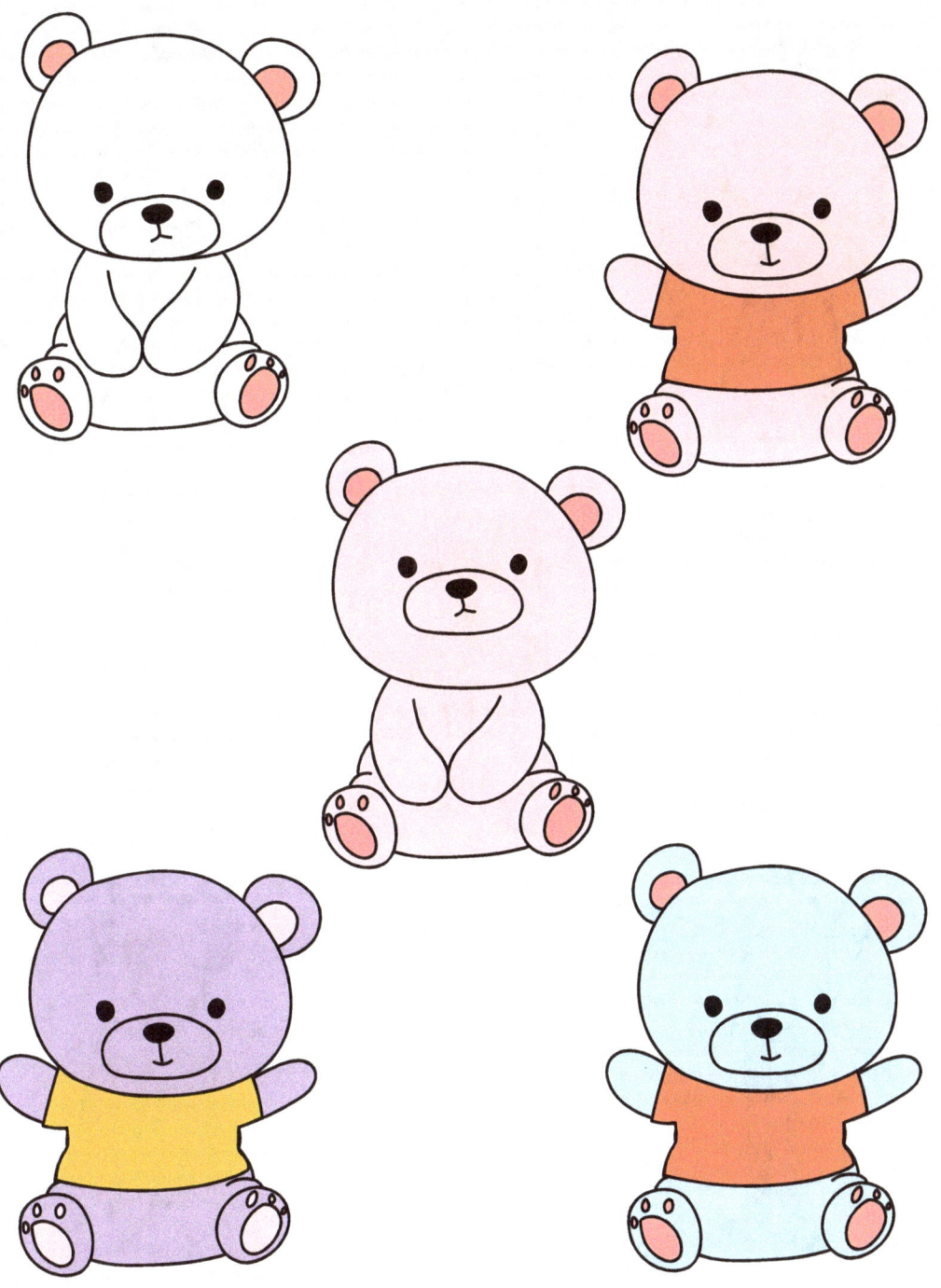

Circle the correct answer.

Circle the girl with the yellow dress and the green headband.

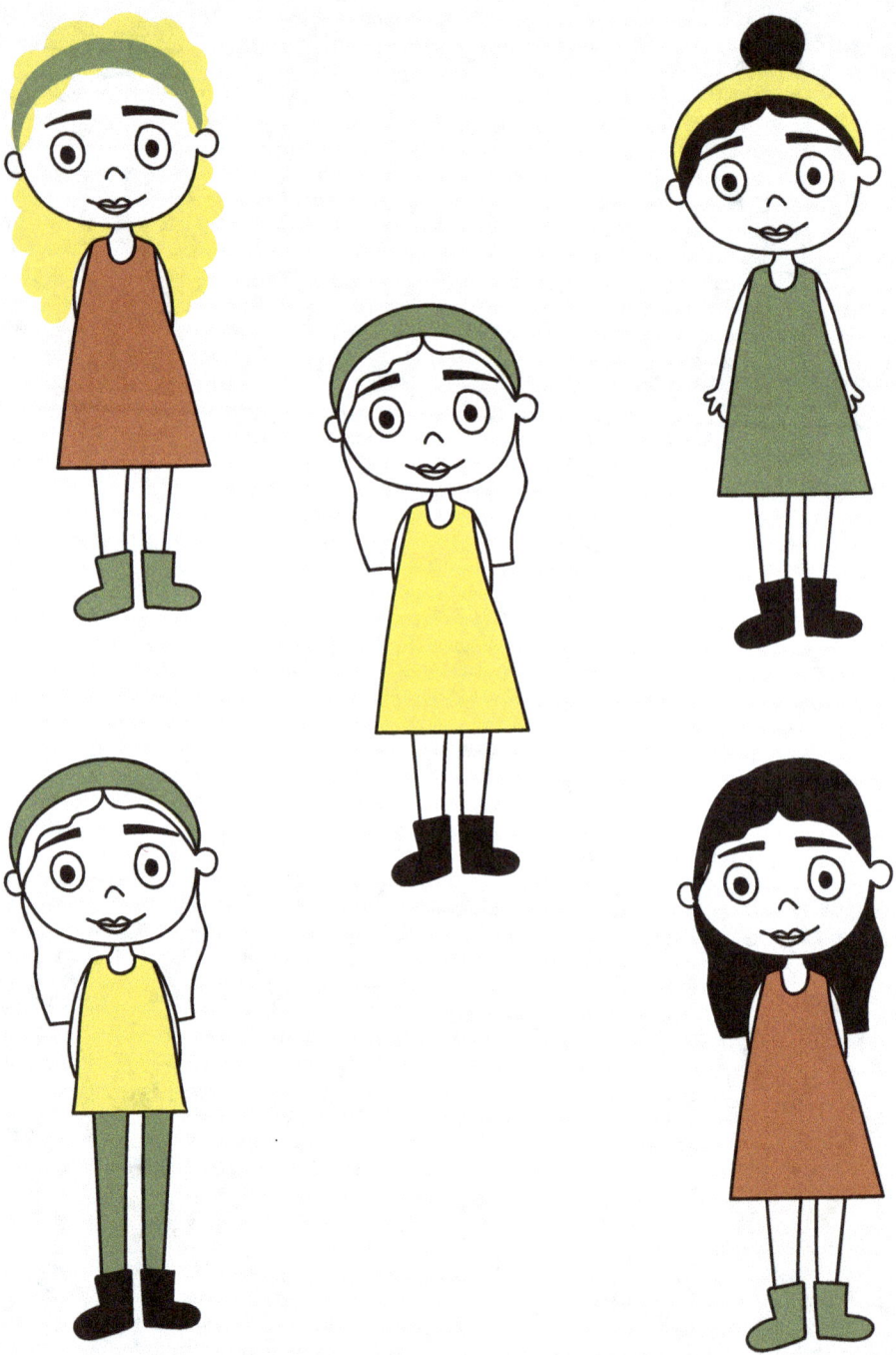

Circle the correct answer.

Circle the house with the black door and blue windows.

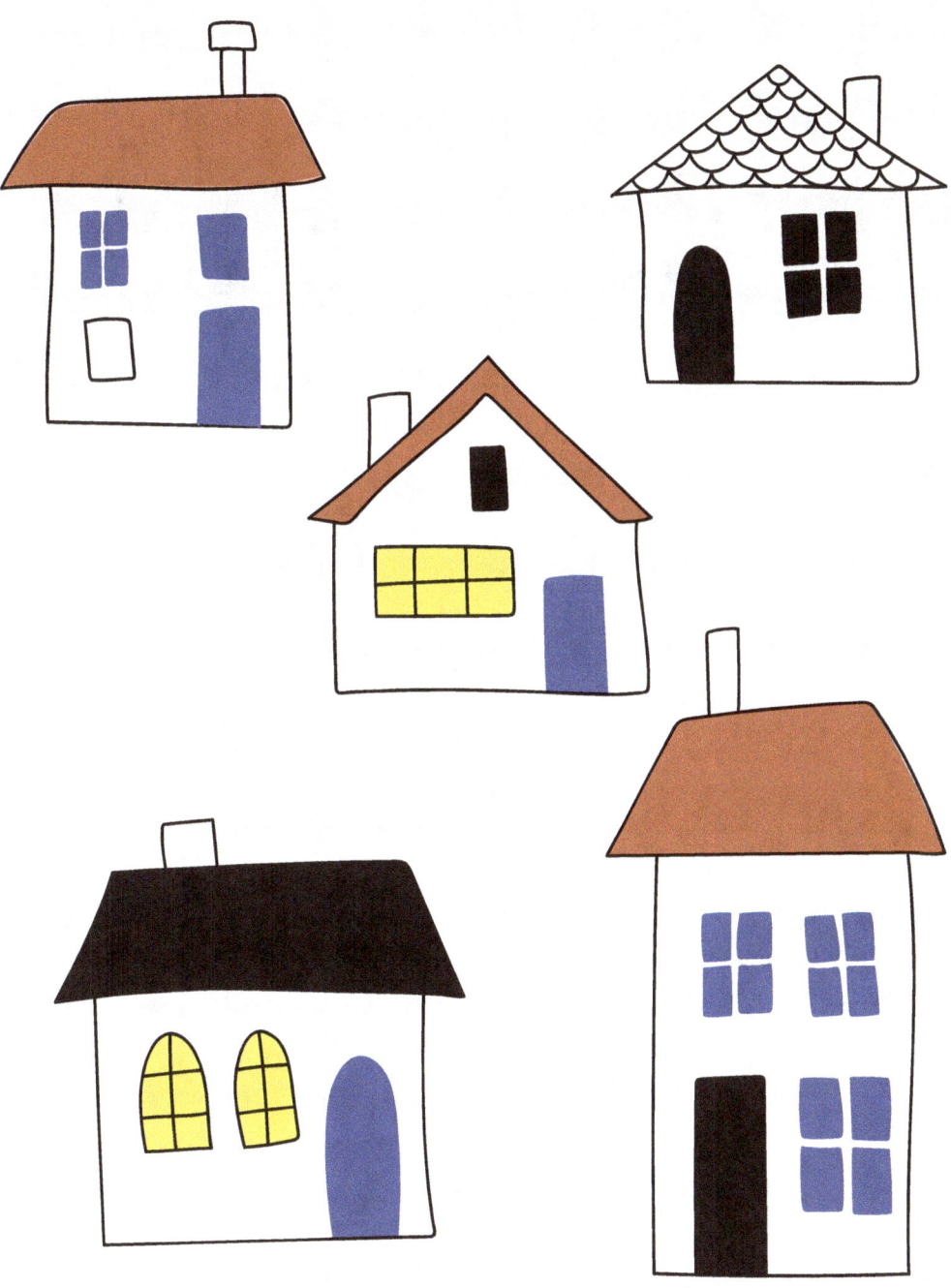

Circle the correct answer.

Circle the fridge that has two cartons of milk and a piece of cheese.

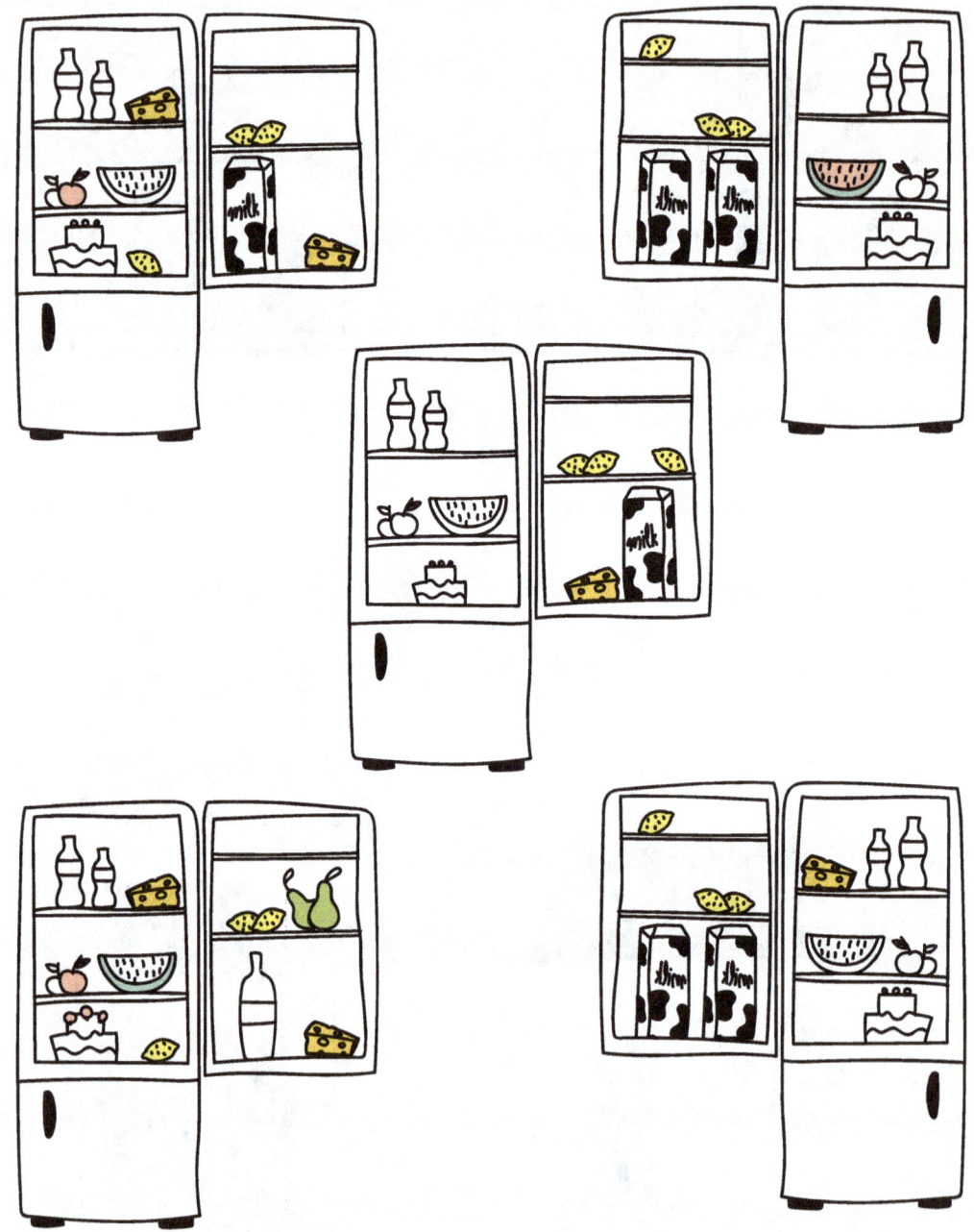

Circle the correct answer.

Circle the pencil case that has only colored pencils.

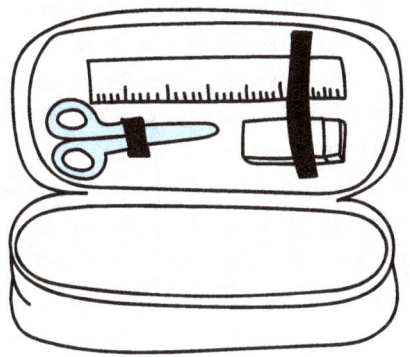 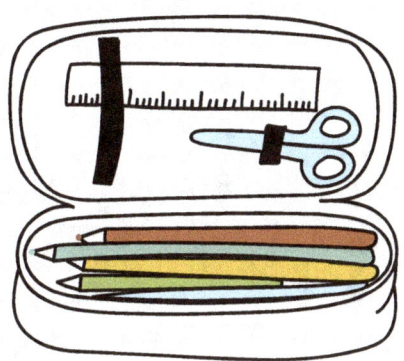

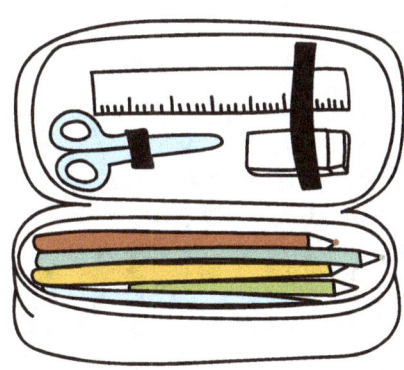

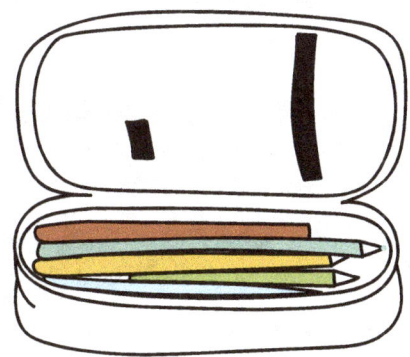 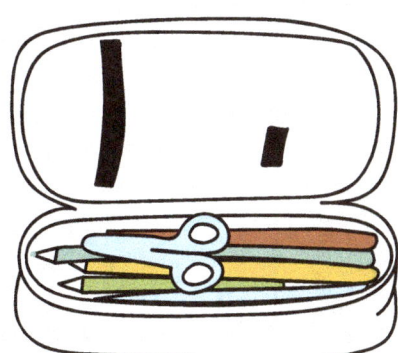

Circle the correct answer.

Circle the bag that has only toys.

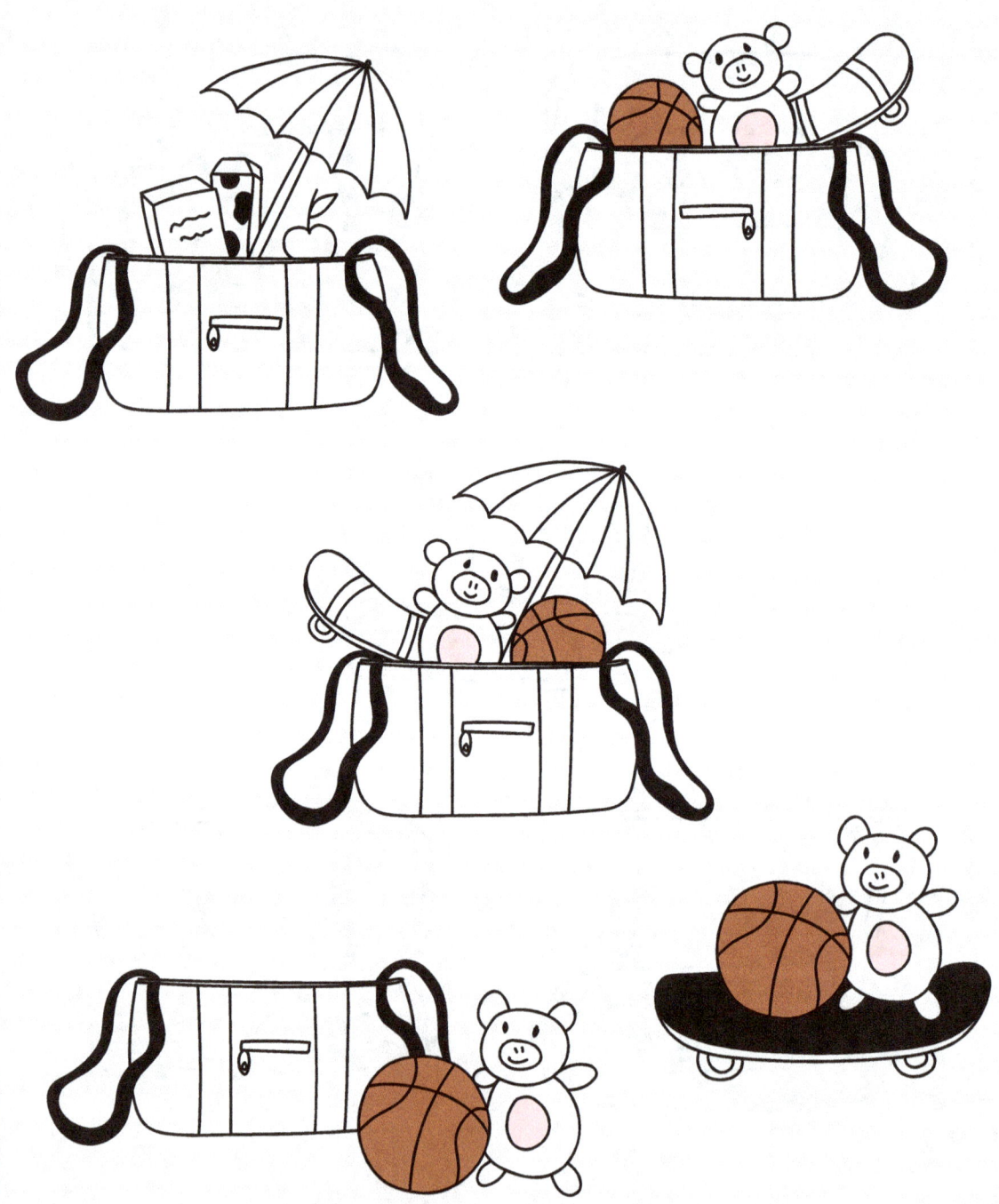

Circle the correct answer.

Circle the boat with three children and two cats.

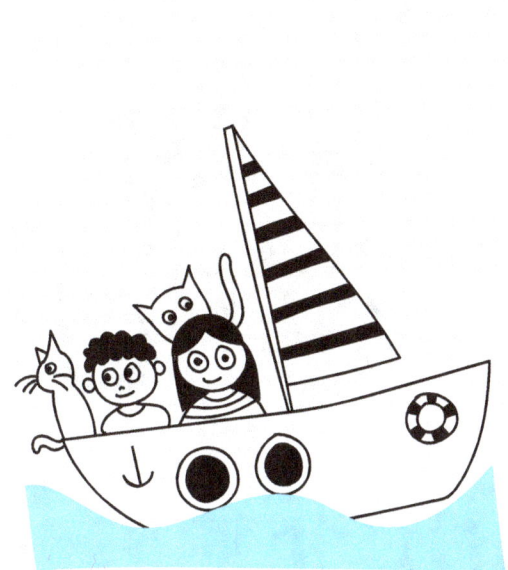

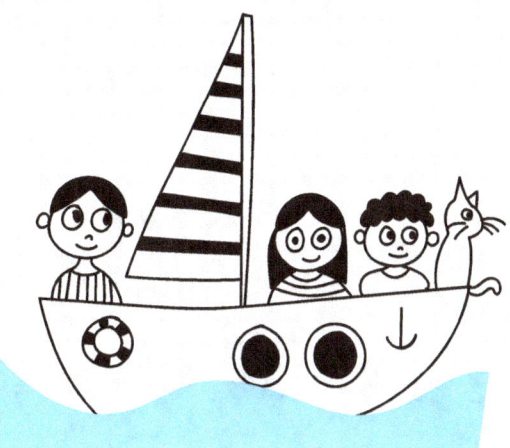

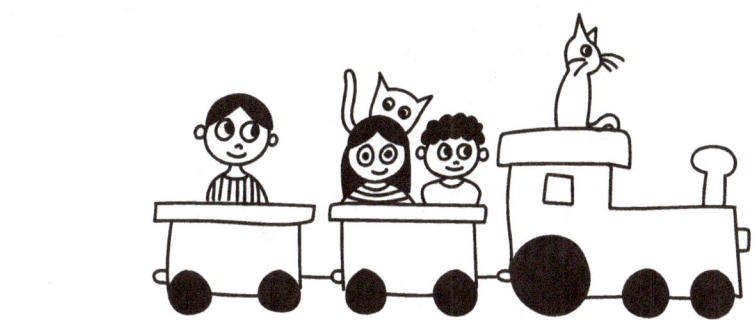

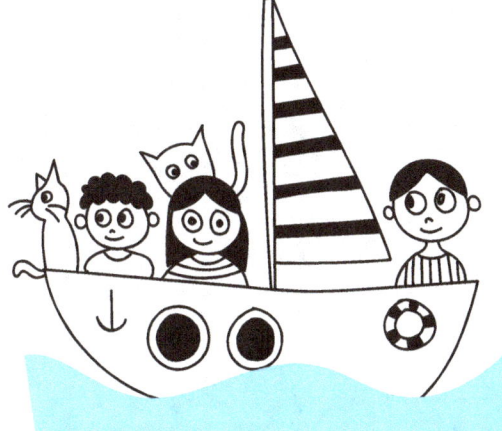

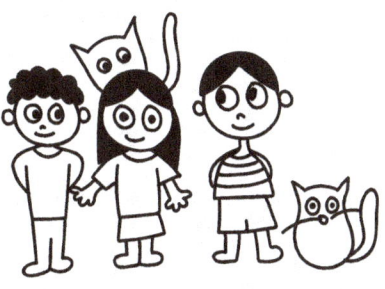

Circle the correct answer.

Circle the car with two little children in it.

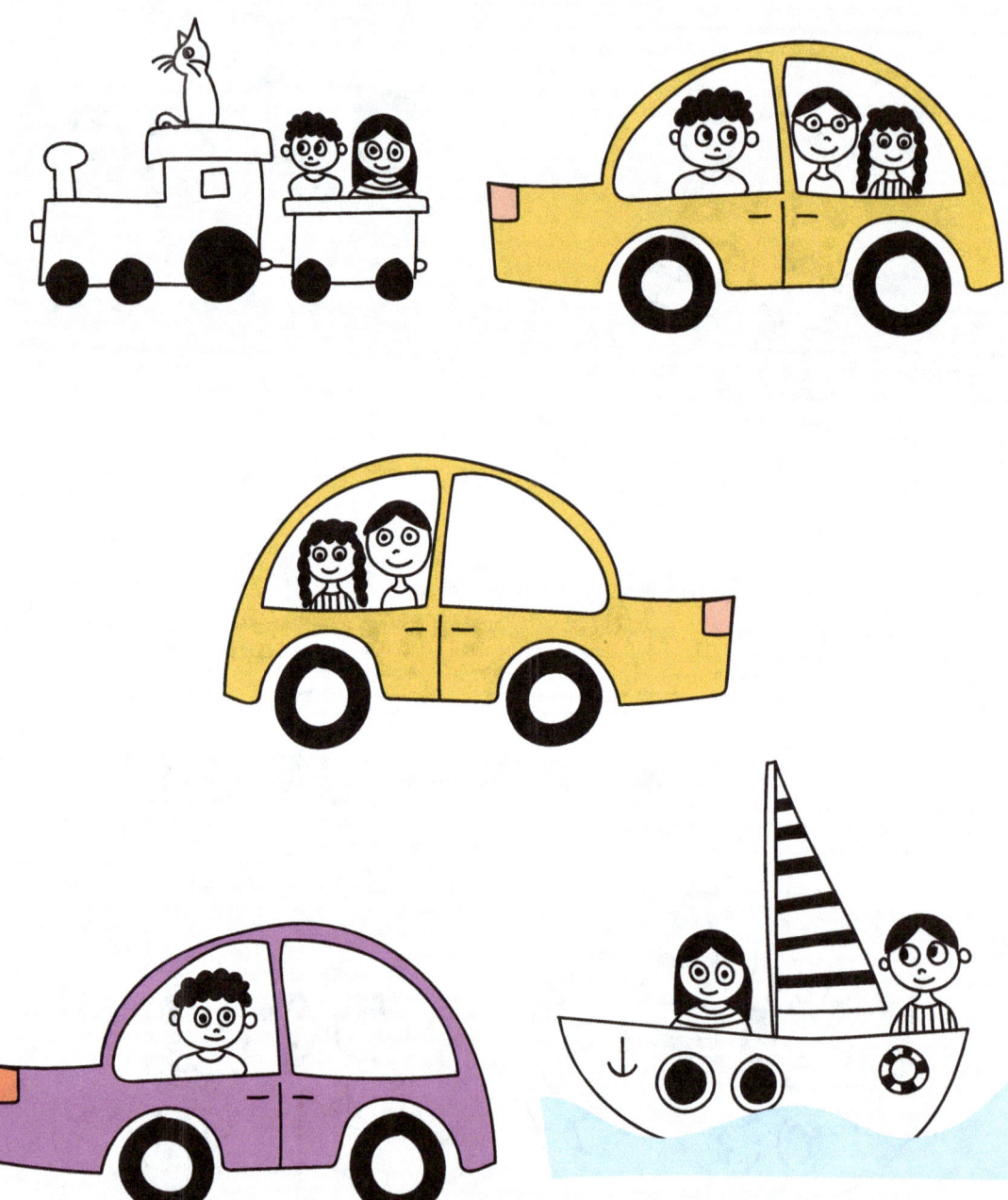

Circle the correct answer.

Circle the rainbow that has only two colors.

Circle the correct answer.

Circle the little green ball.

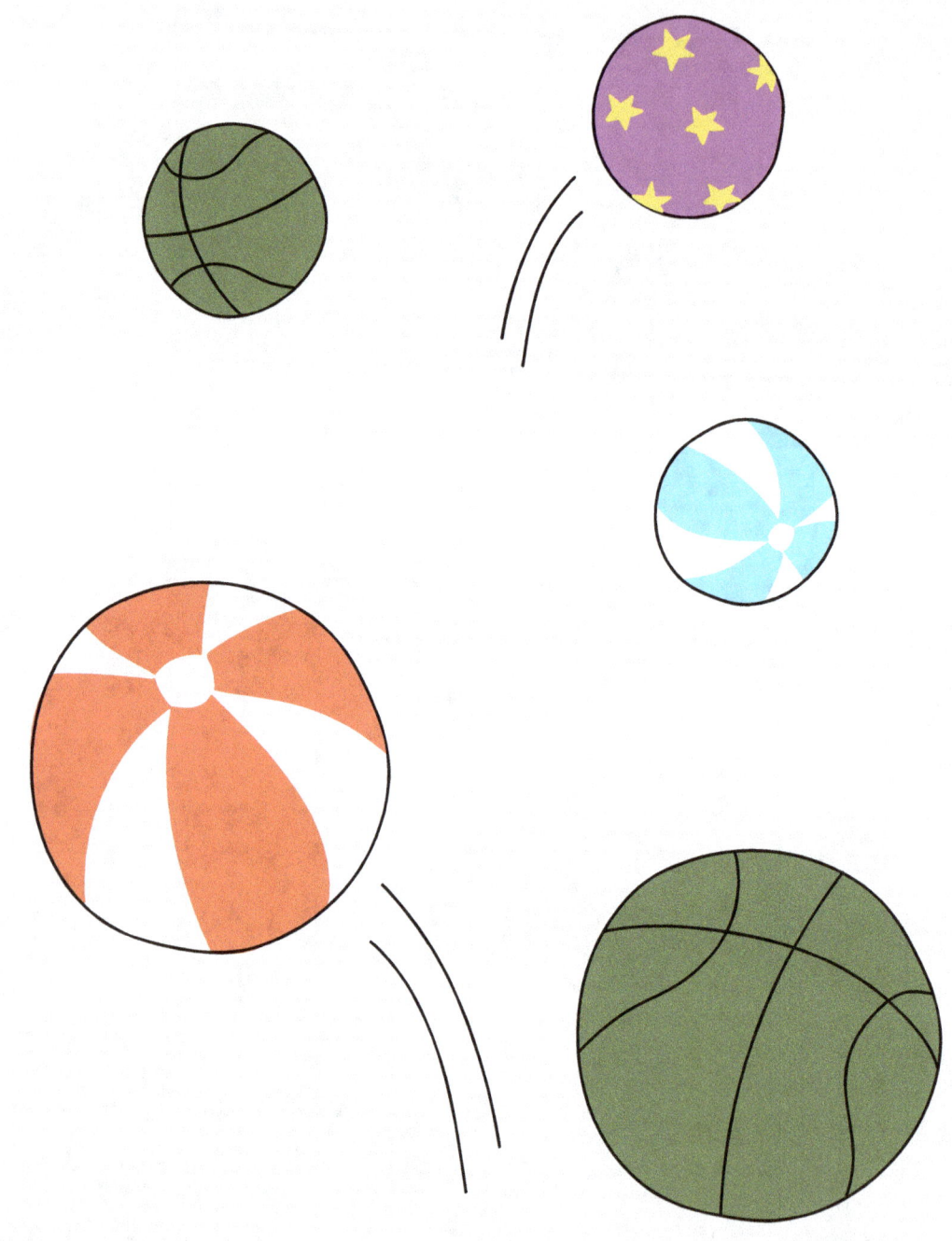

Circle the correct answer.

Circle the black box containing three balls.

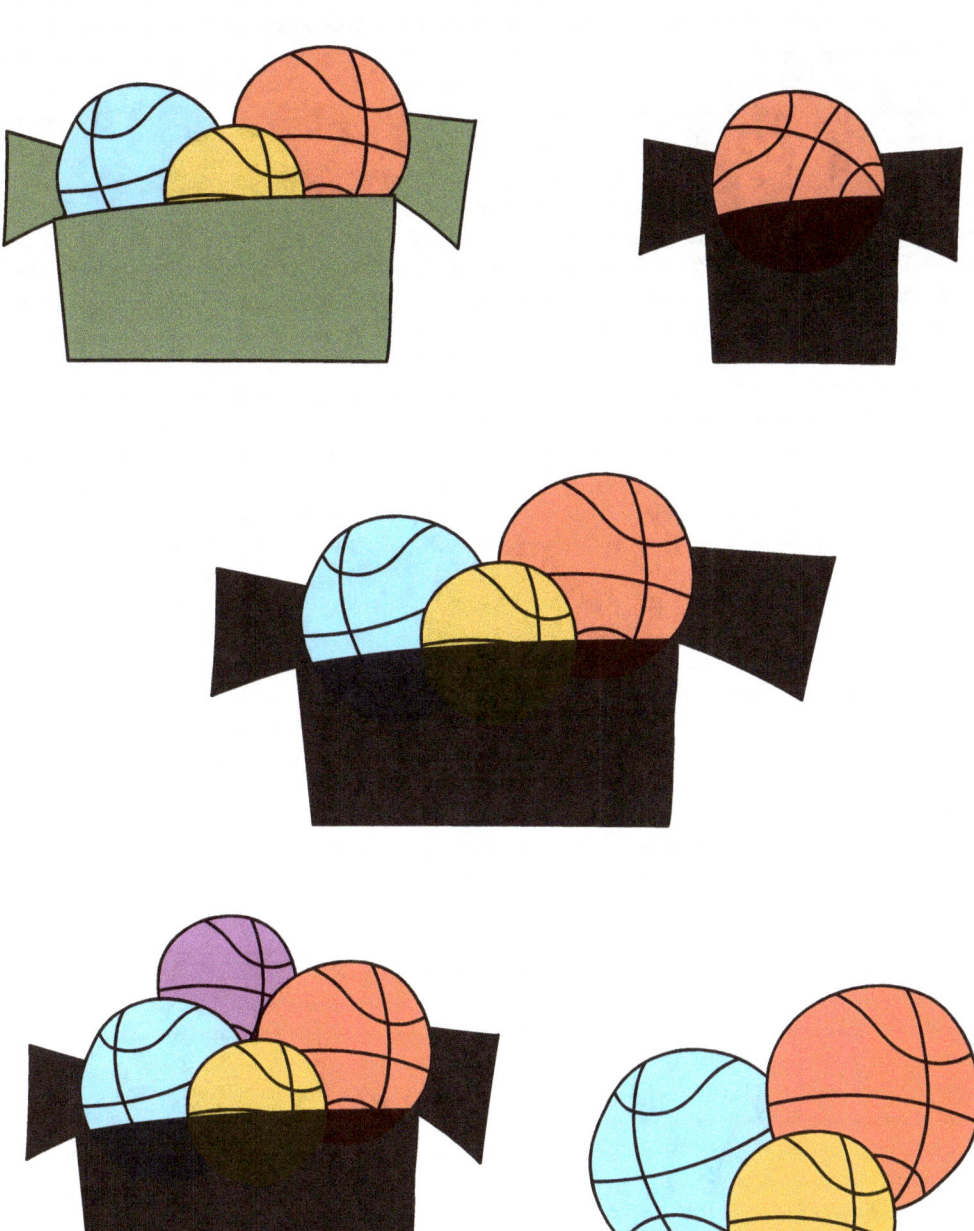

Circle the correct answer.

Circle the long trousers with pockets.

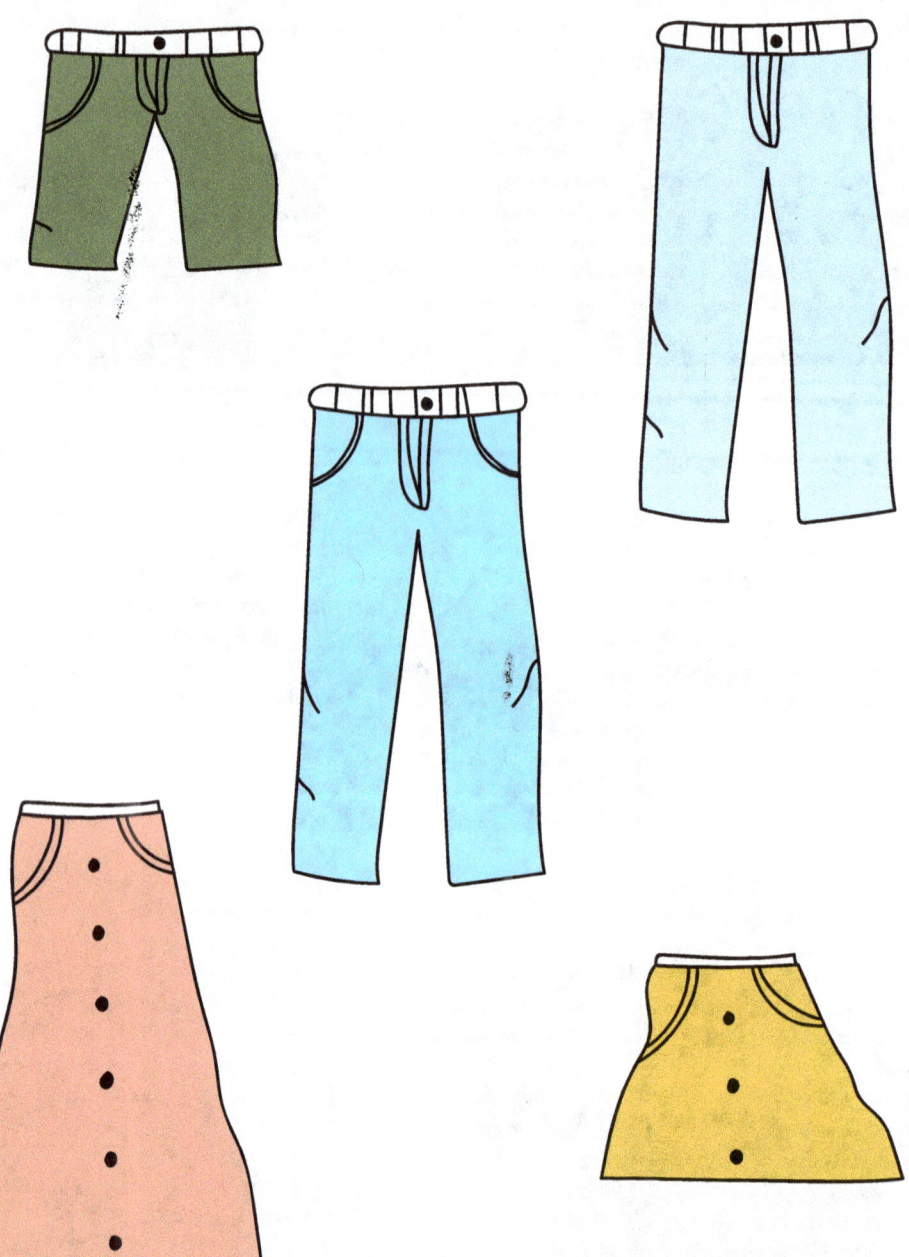

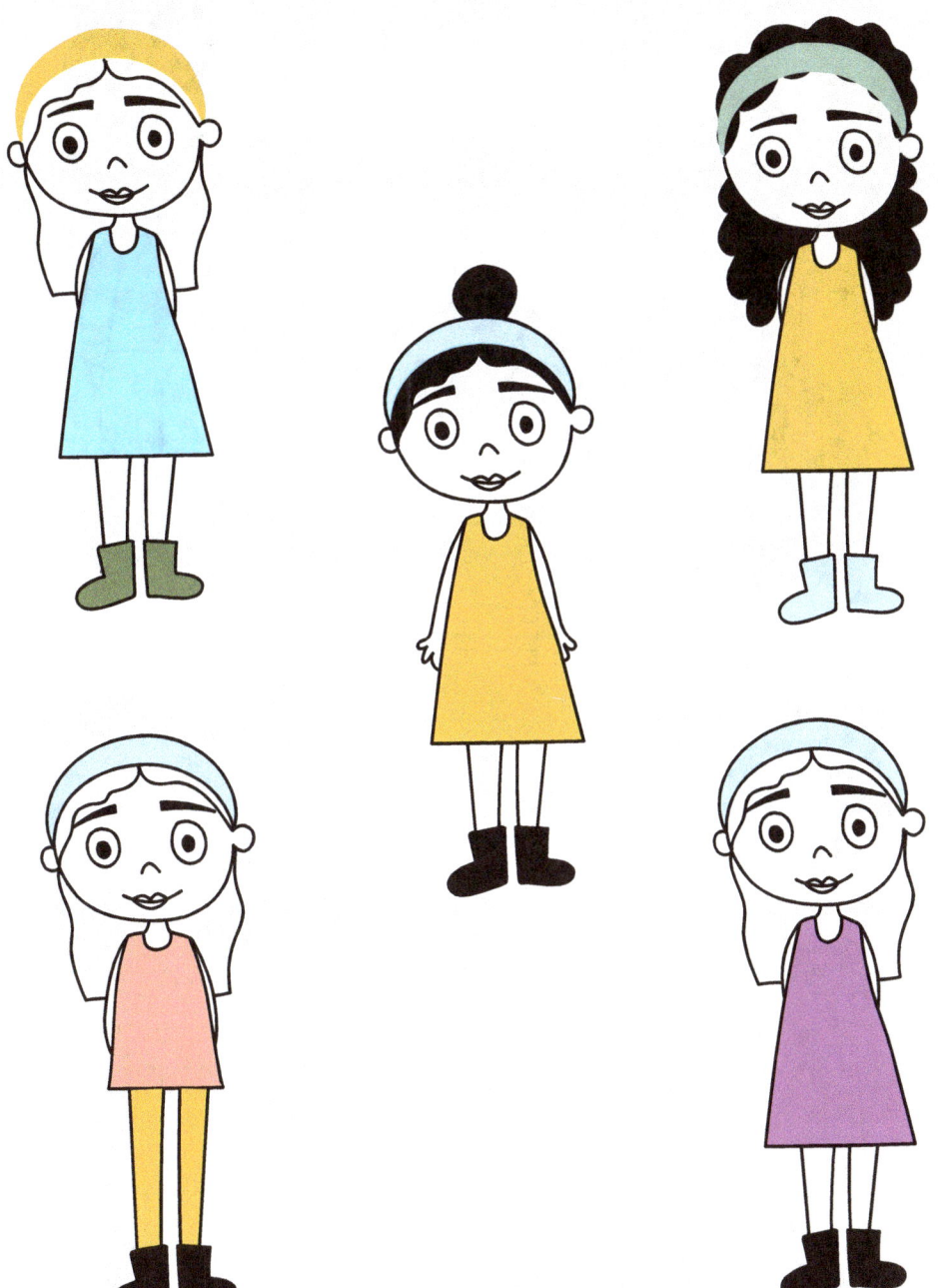

Circle the correct answer.

Circle the girl who is wearing an orange dress and a blue headband.

Circle the correct answer.

Circle the boy wearing summer clothes.

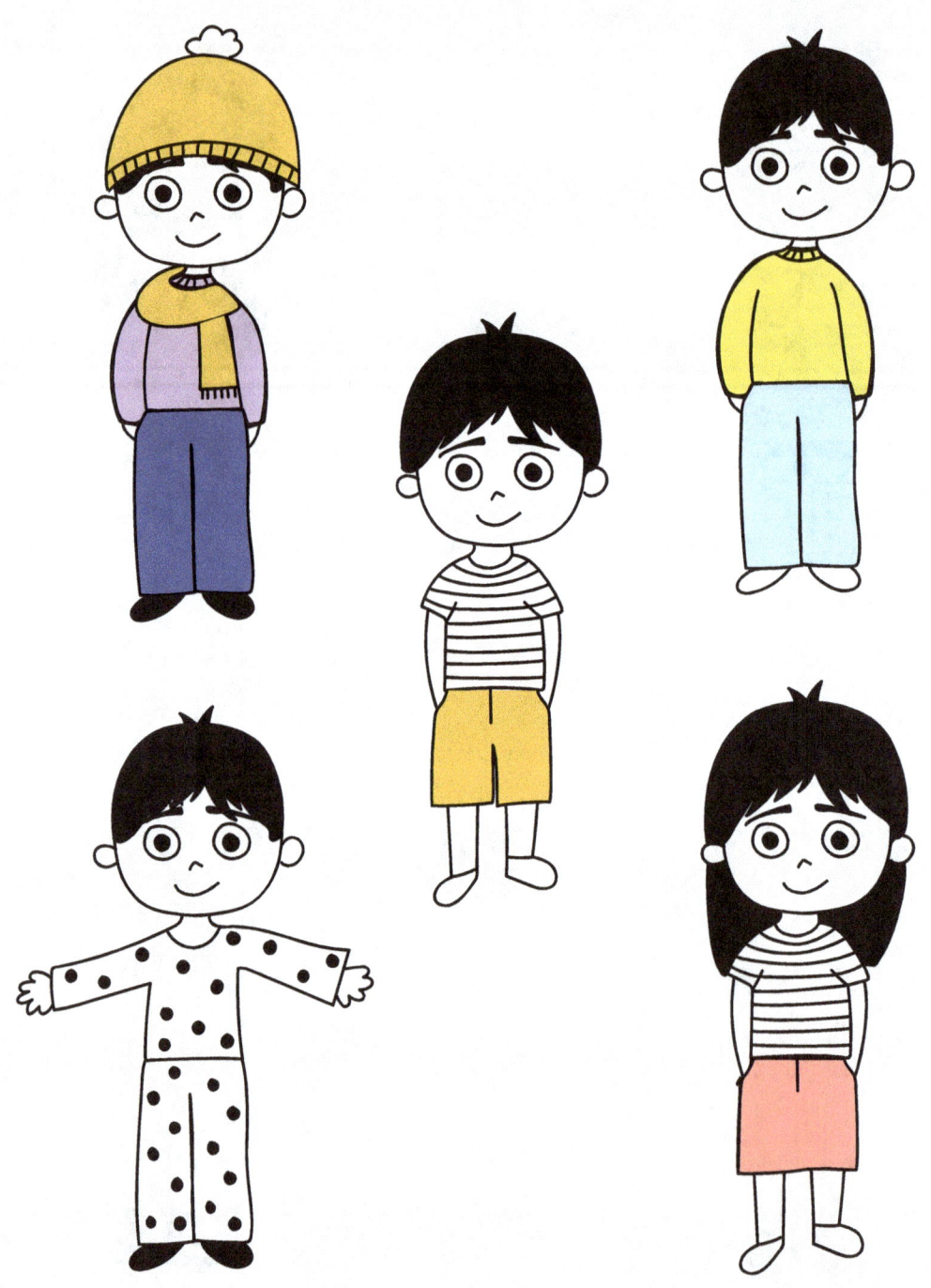

Circle the correct answer.

Circle the pond that has four little frogs.

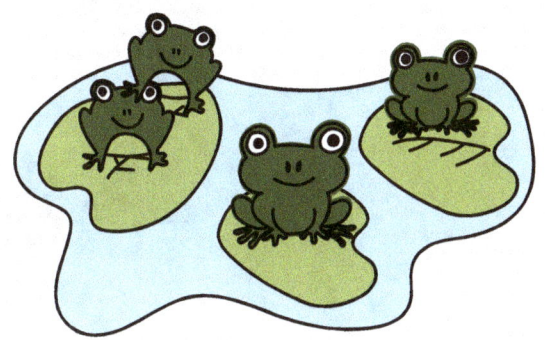
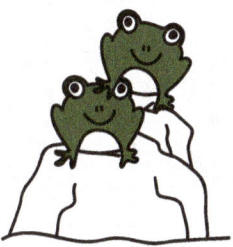

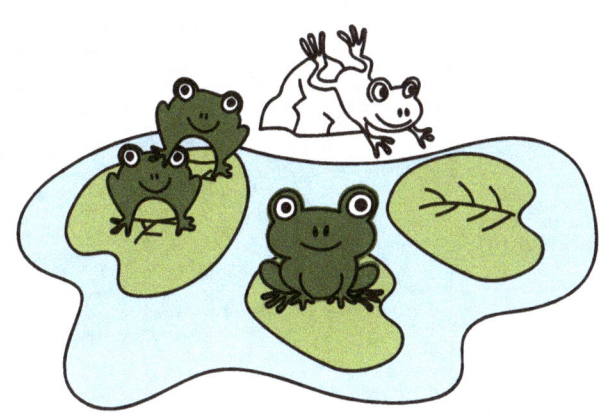

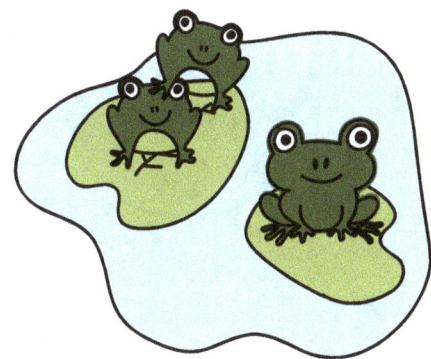
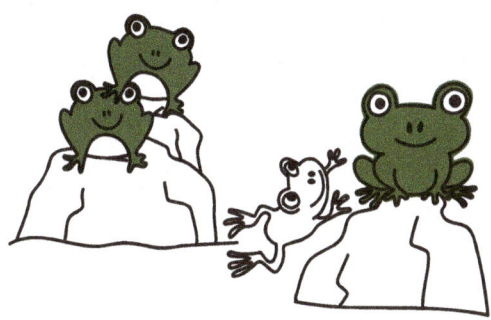

Circle the correct answer.

Circle the meadow with the cows.

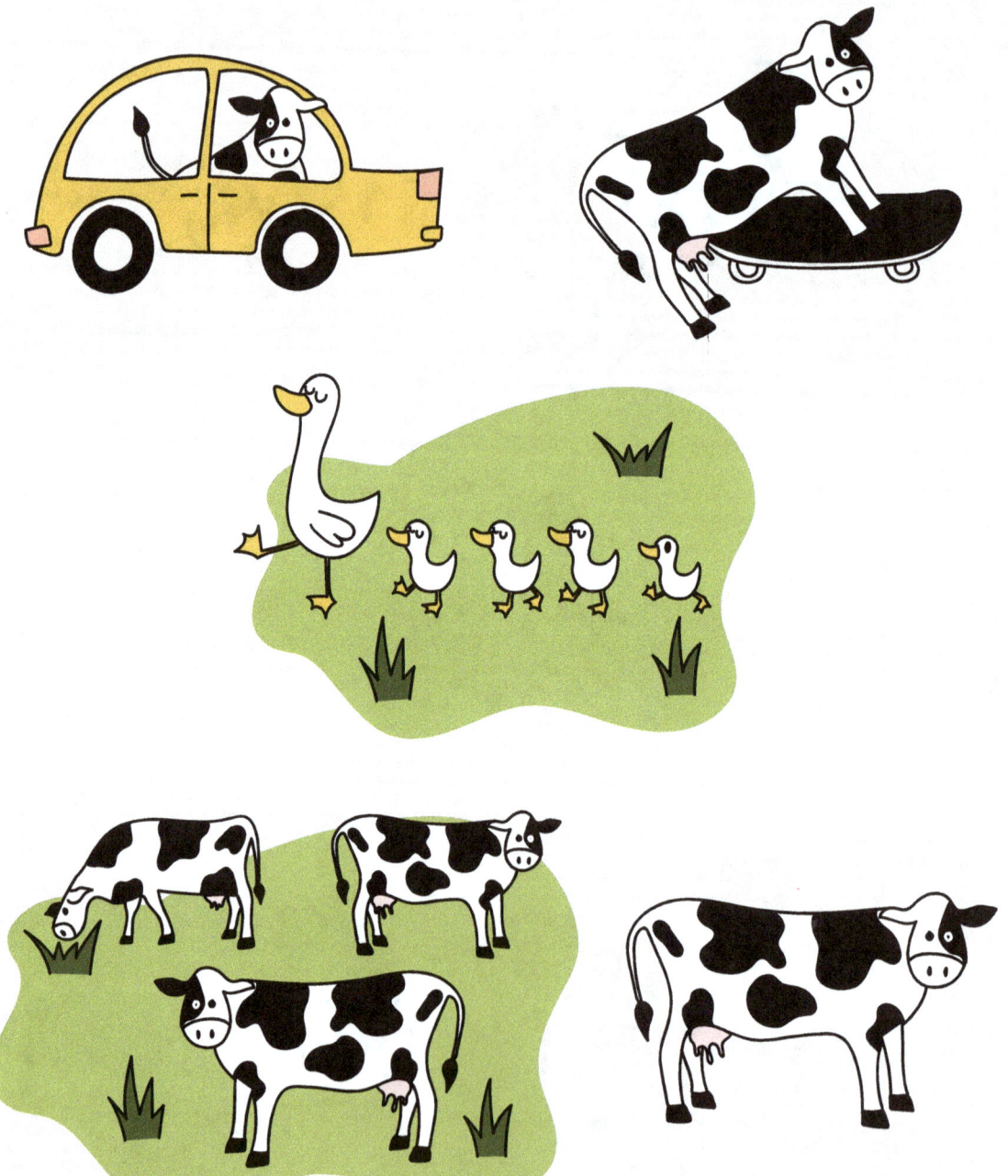

Circle the correct answer.

Circle the family with the fewest children.

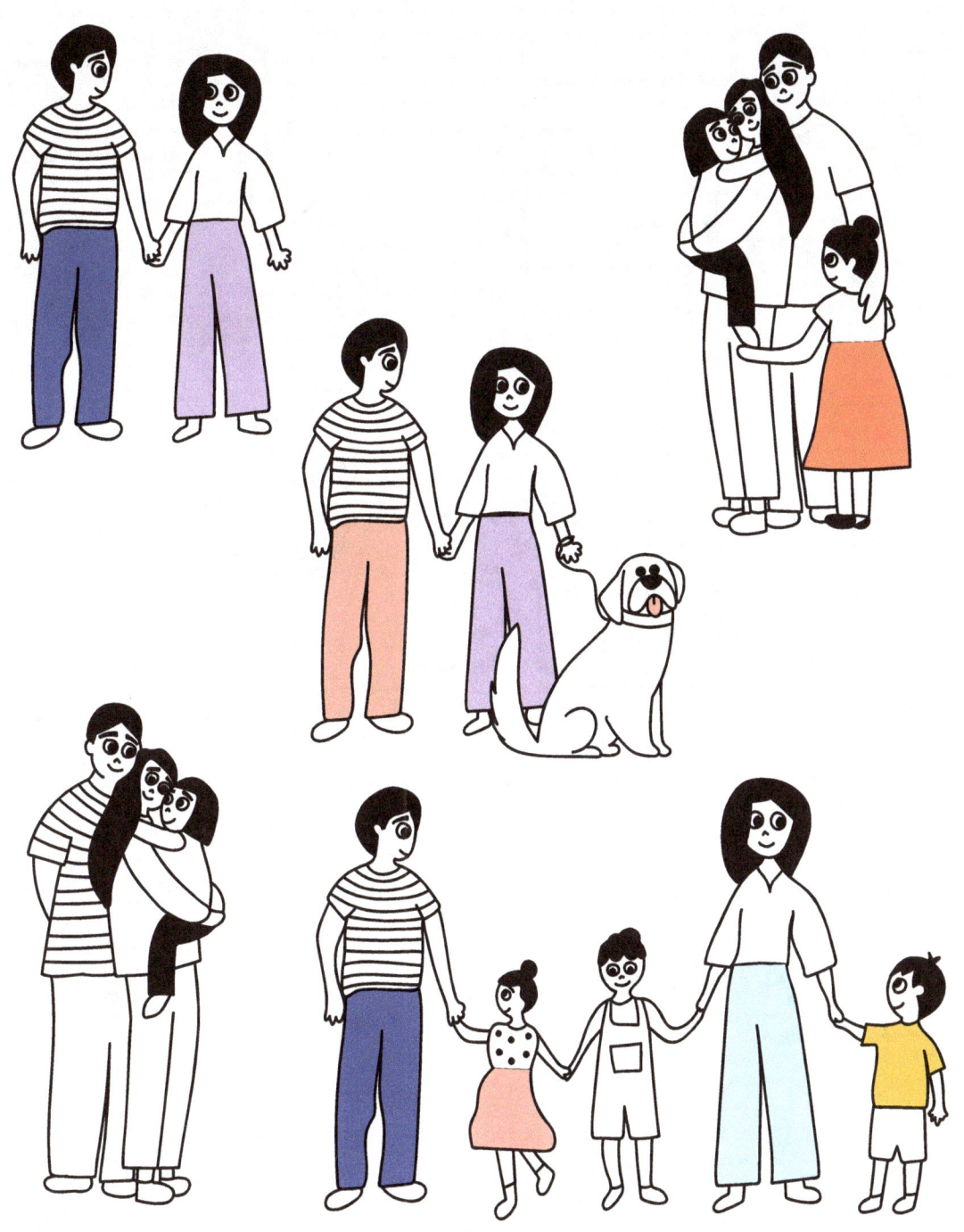

Circle the correct answer.

Circle the park that has three swings.

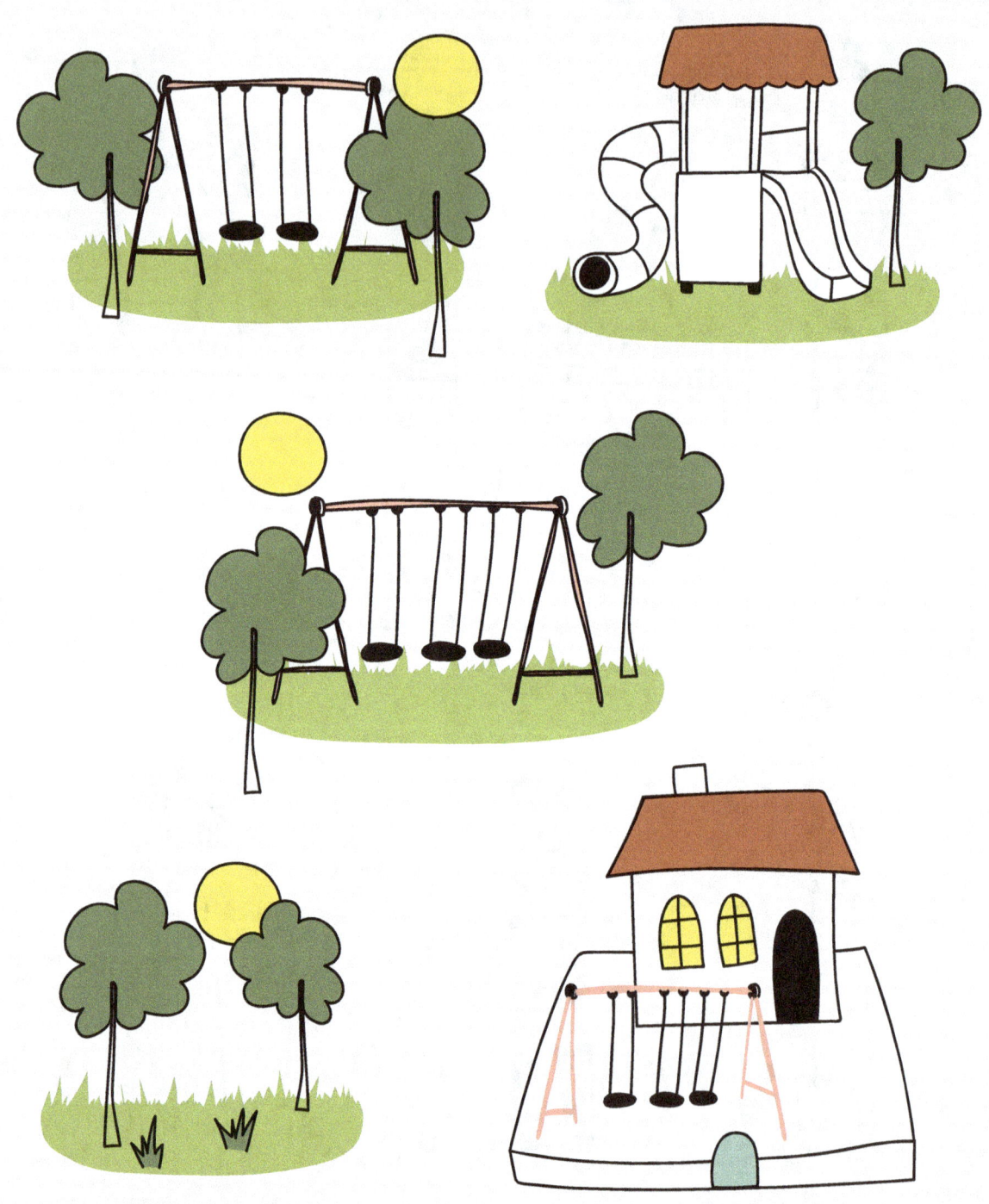

Circle the correct answer.

Circle the puppy with the brown spots.

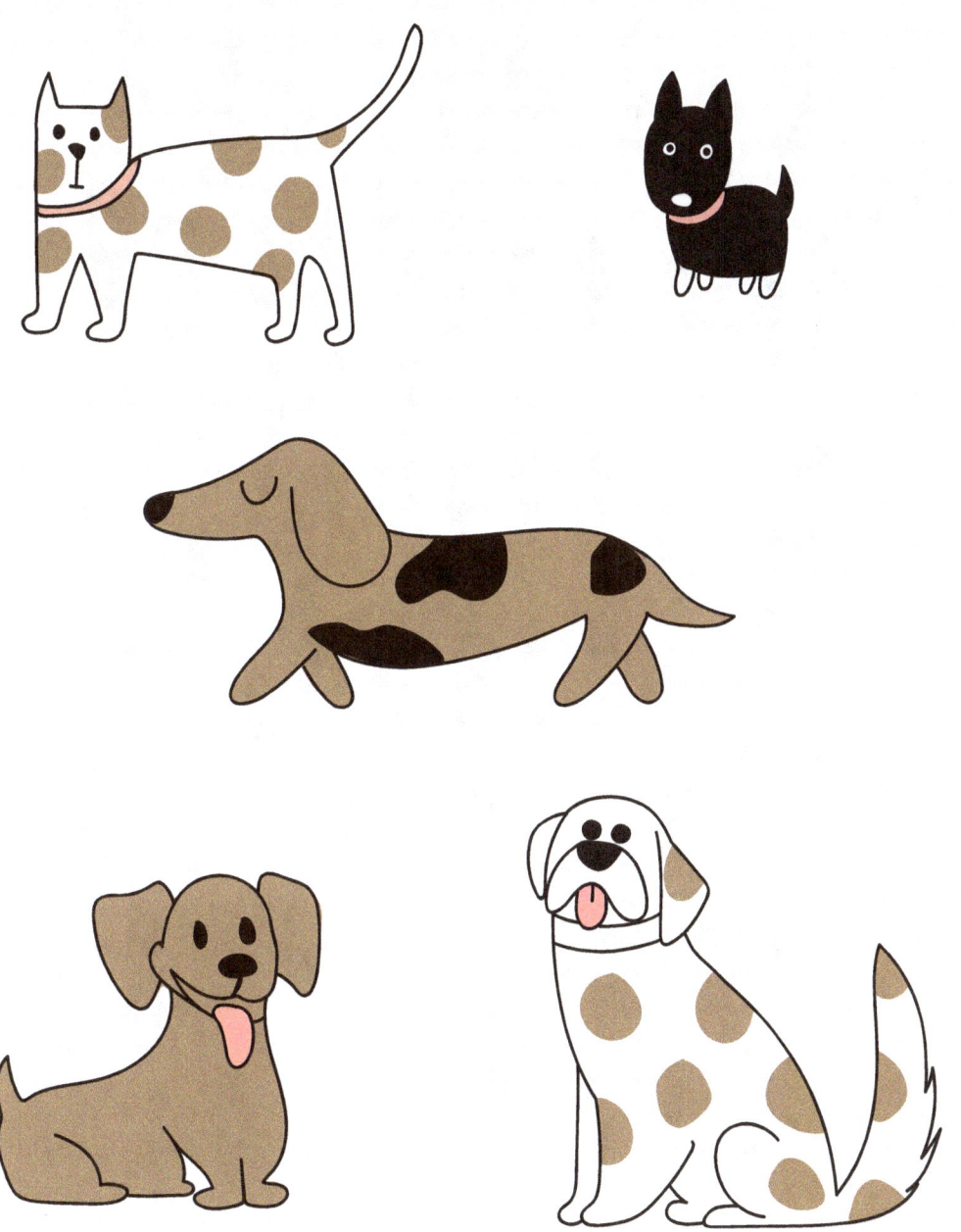

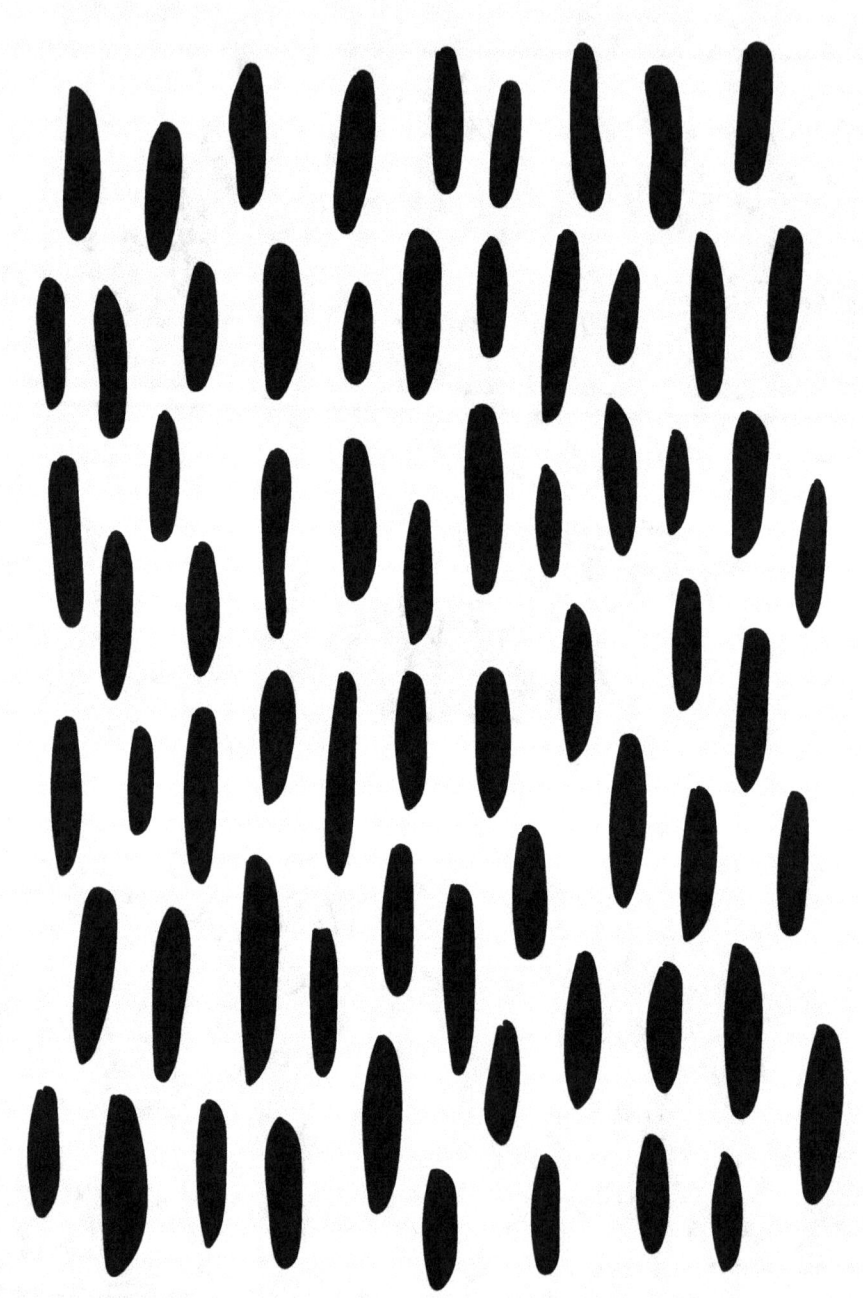

LEVEL 2

Color the picture following the instructions.

In the brown vase, there are six flowers. Two of the flowers are yellow, one is red and three are pink.

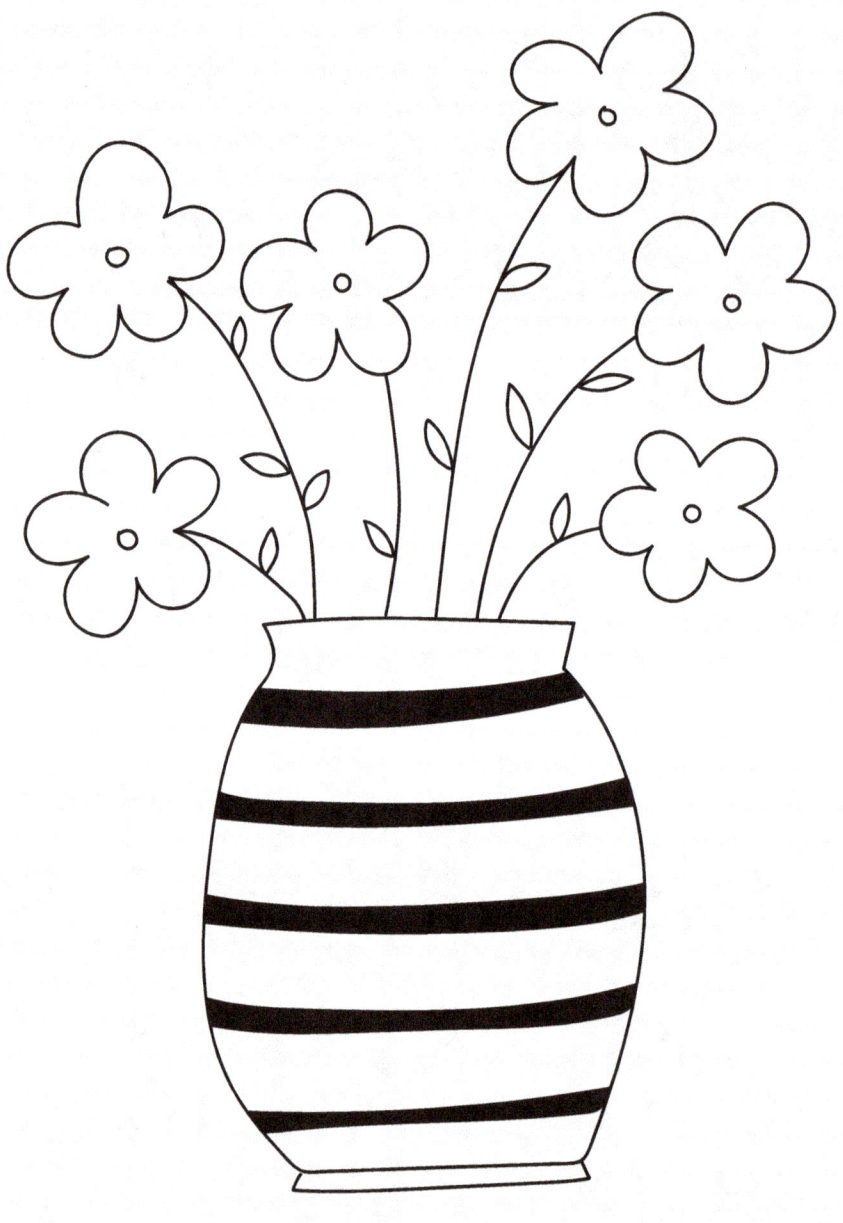

Color the picture following the instructions.

There are four different fruits in the red fruit jar: a yellow apple, a green lemon, a yellow melon, and red cherries.

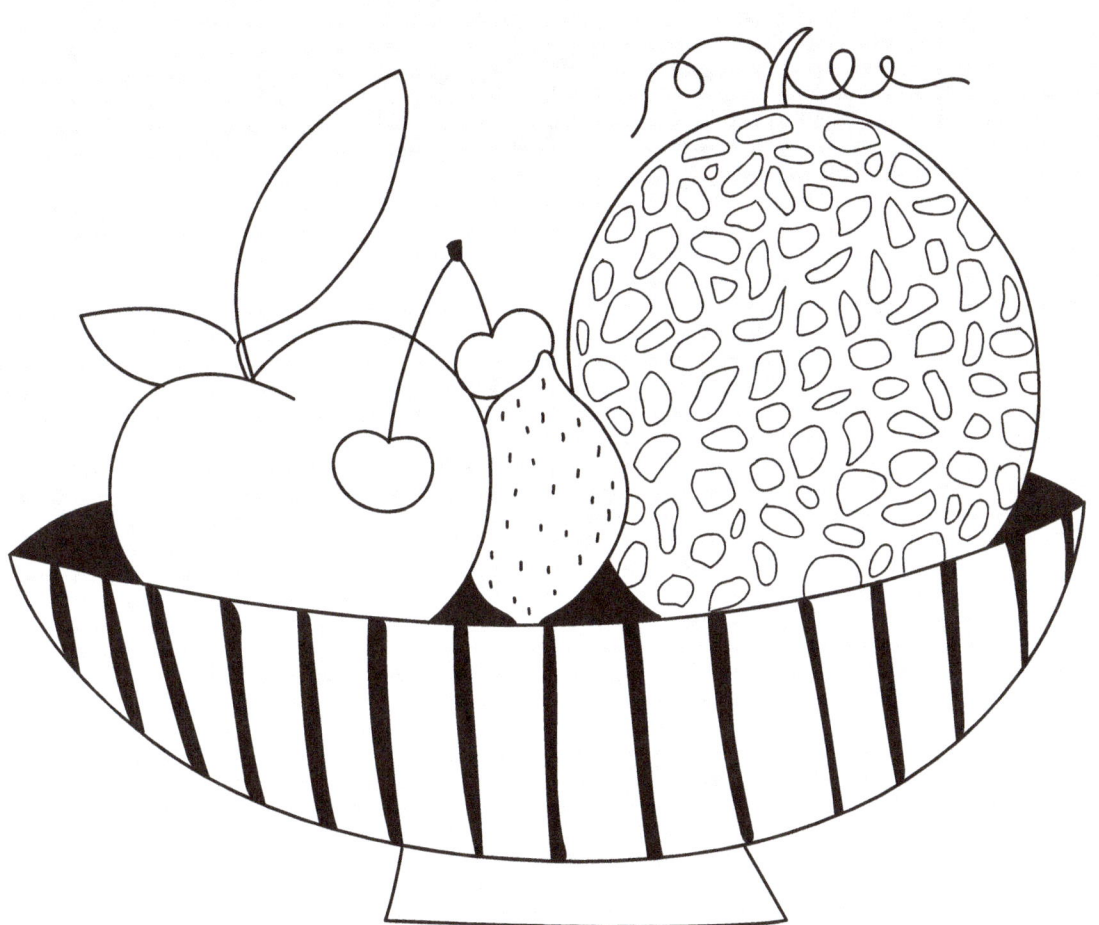

Color the picture following the instructions.

Mary's hair is brown. She has two big blue eyes and cherry-red lips! She is wearing her favorite pink dress, and the butterfly on her dress is yellow. She wears a yellow headband and brown shoes.

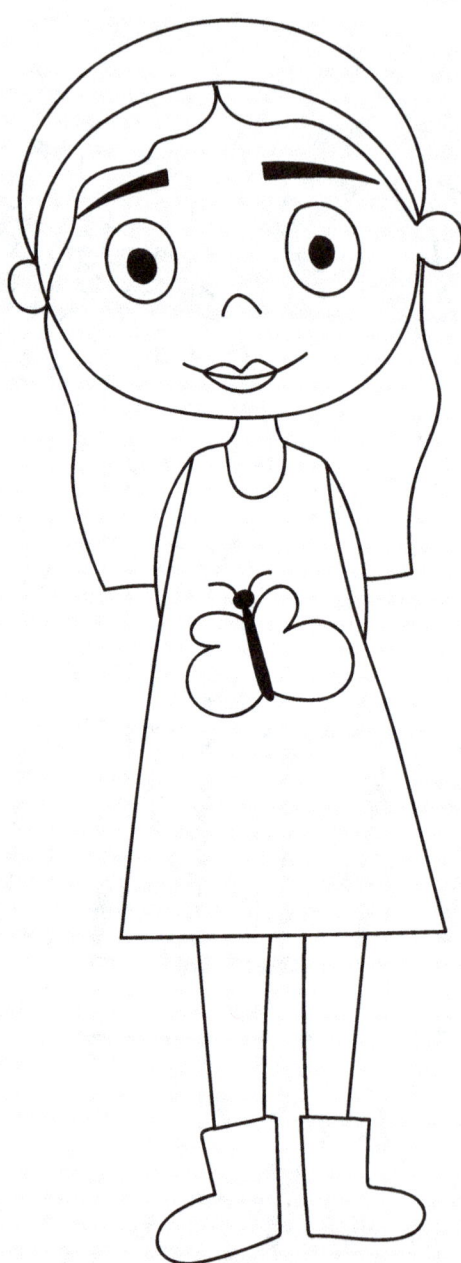

Color the picture following the instructions.

Ben is the big dog with black spots on his back and grey color on his belly, wearing a blue collar. Zuzu is the small dog. She is black with white paws and wears a pink collar. The little kitty is brown with an orange tail and a red collar.

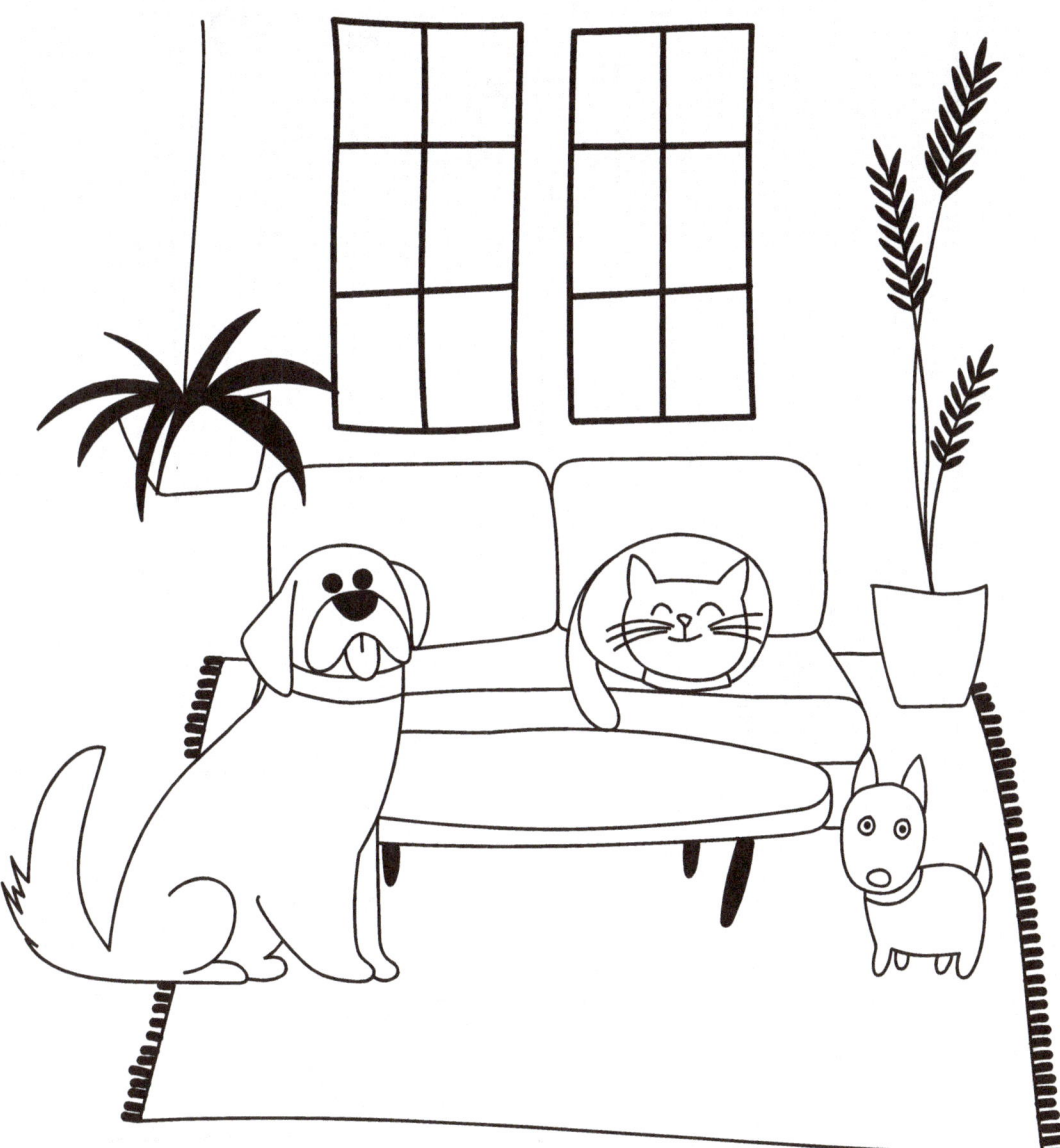

Color the picture following the instructions.

In the closet, there are two pink dresses and a blue one, a pair of brown trousers and a black coat.

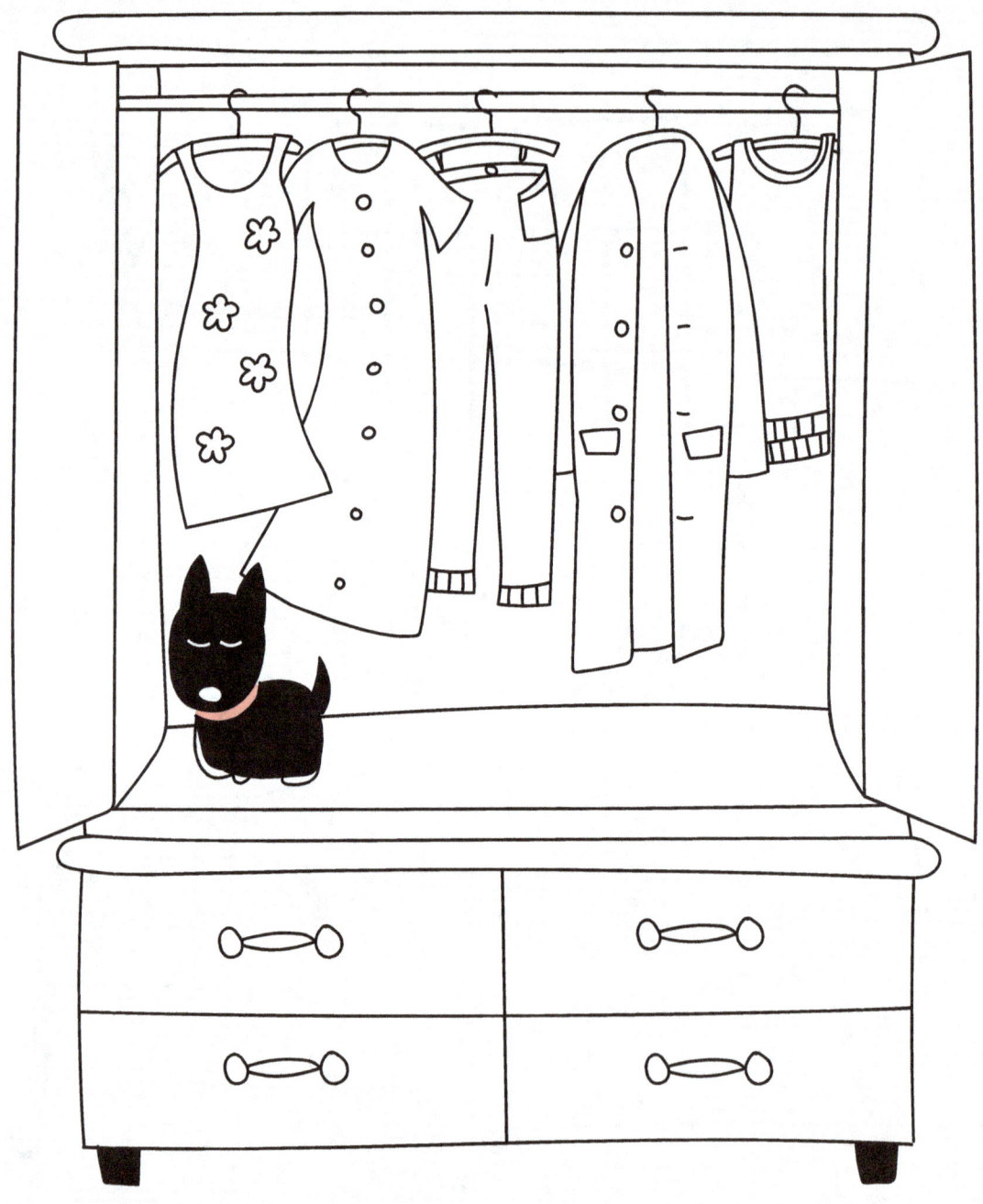

Color the picture following the instructions.

Dad has black hair and black eyes. He is wearing a light blue shirt and blue trousers. His tie is grey, and he wears black shoes. Mom has red hair and brown eyes. She is wearing an orange skirt with a white blouse and orange shoes. Little George has the same hair color as Dad and the same eye color as Mom. He wears blue jeans and a yellow T-shirt.

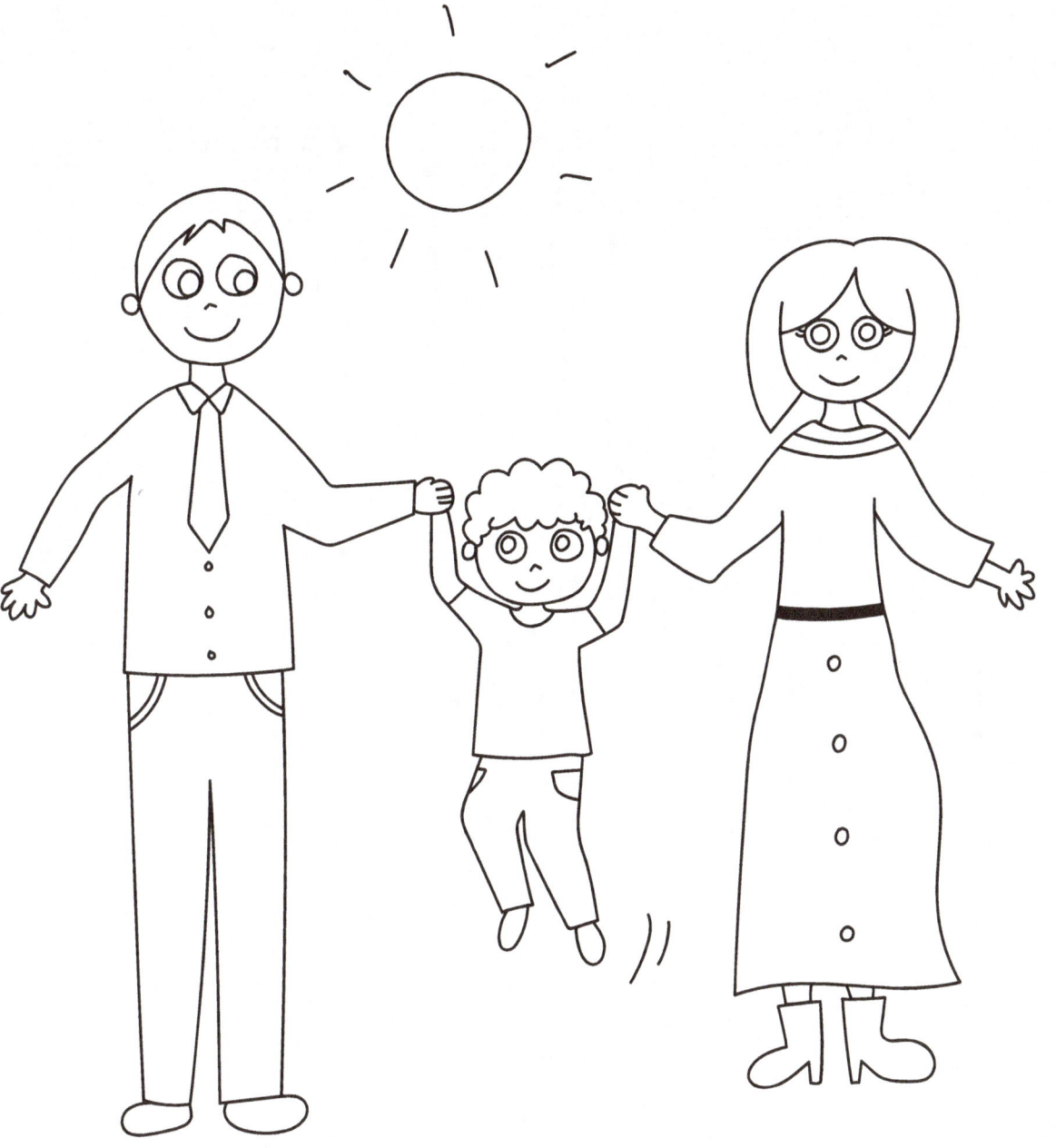

Color the picture following the instructions.

The playground in our neighborhood is very well-equipped. It has a big red slide and a small yellow one. It has three green swings and a blue climbing wall. There is a brown bench where we can sit and rest and a black table with brown chairs where we can eat our snacks.

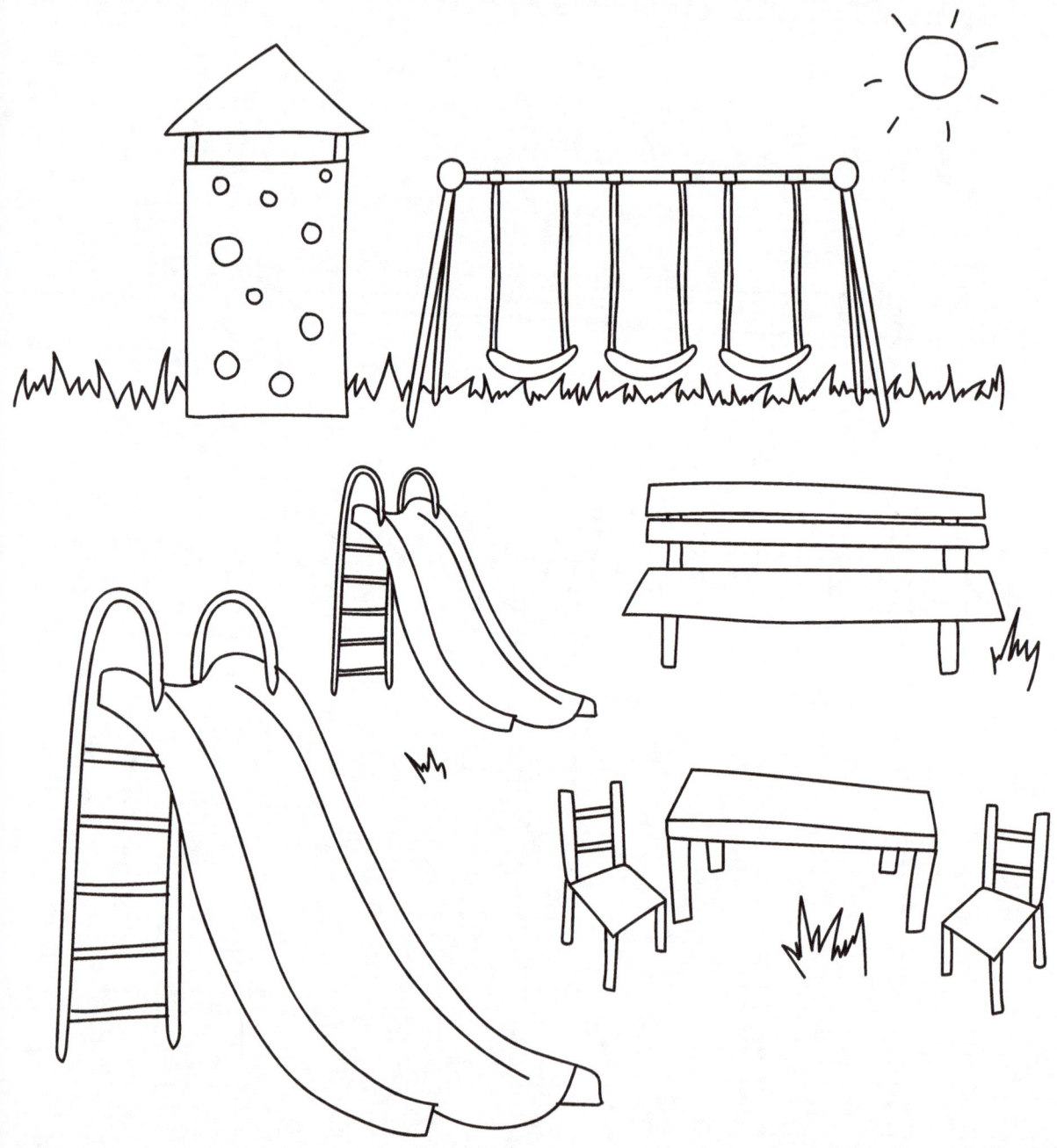

Color the picture following the instructions.

Jenny has the most colorful room in the world. Her bed is pink, and her bookcase is purple. She has a small blue bedside table and a big brown dresser. Her desk is green with brown stripes, and her desk chair is red. Jenny's room has all the colors of the rainbow!

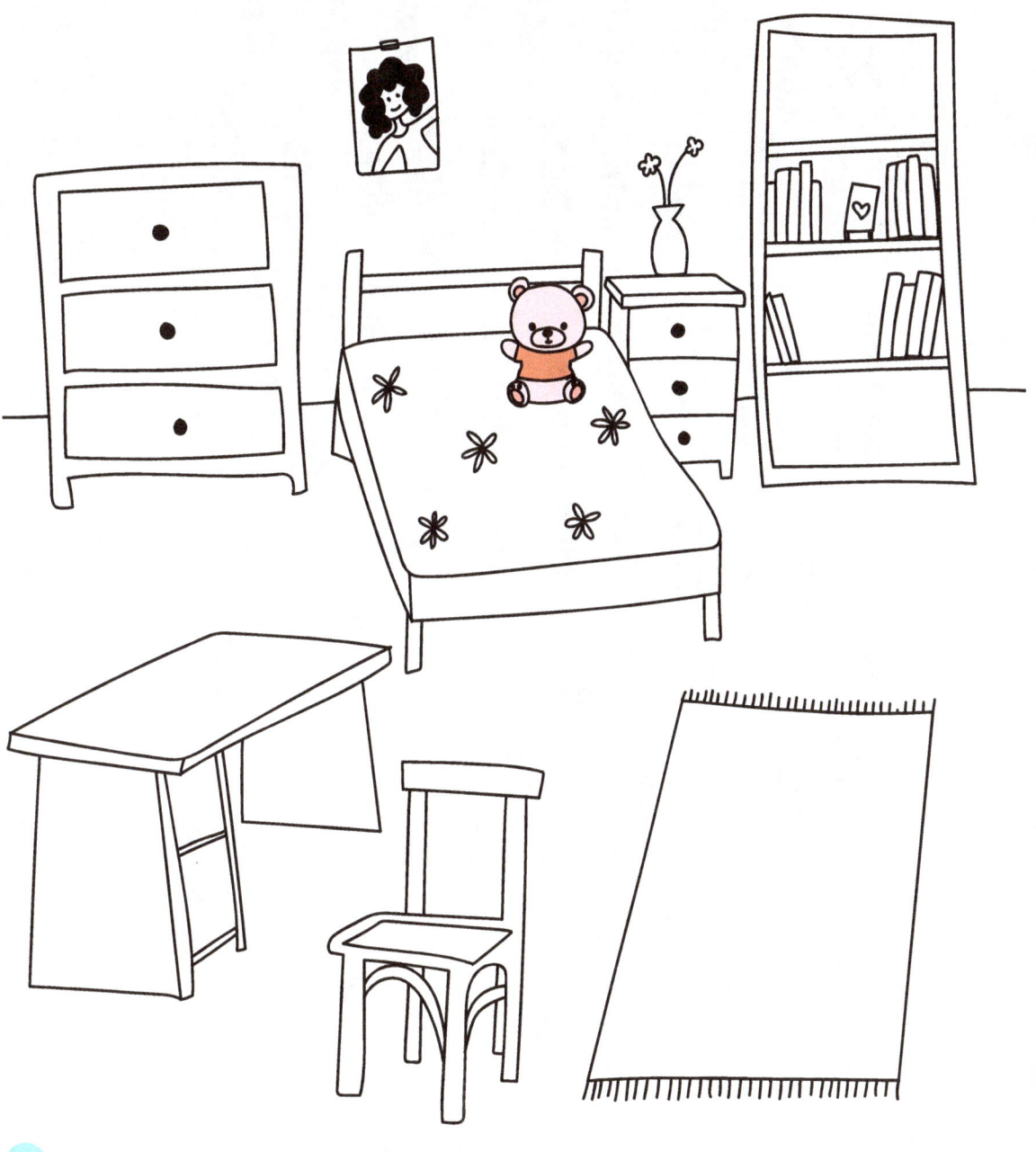

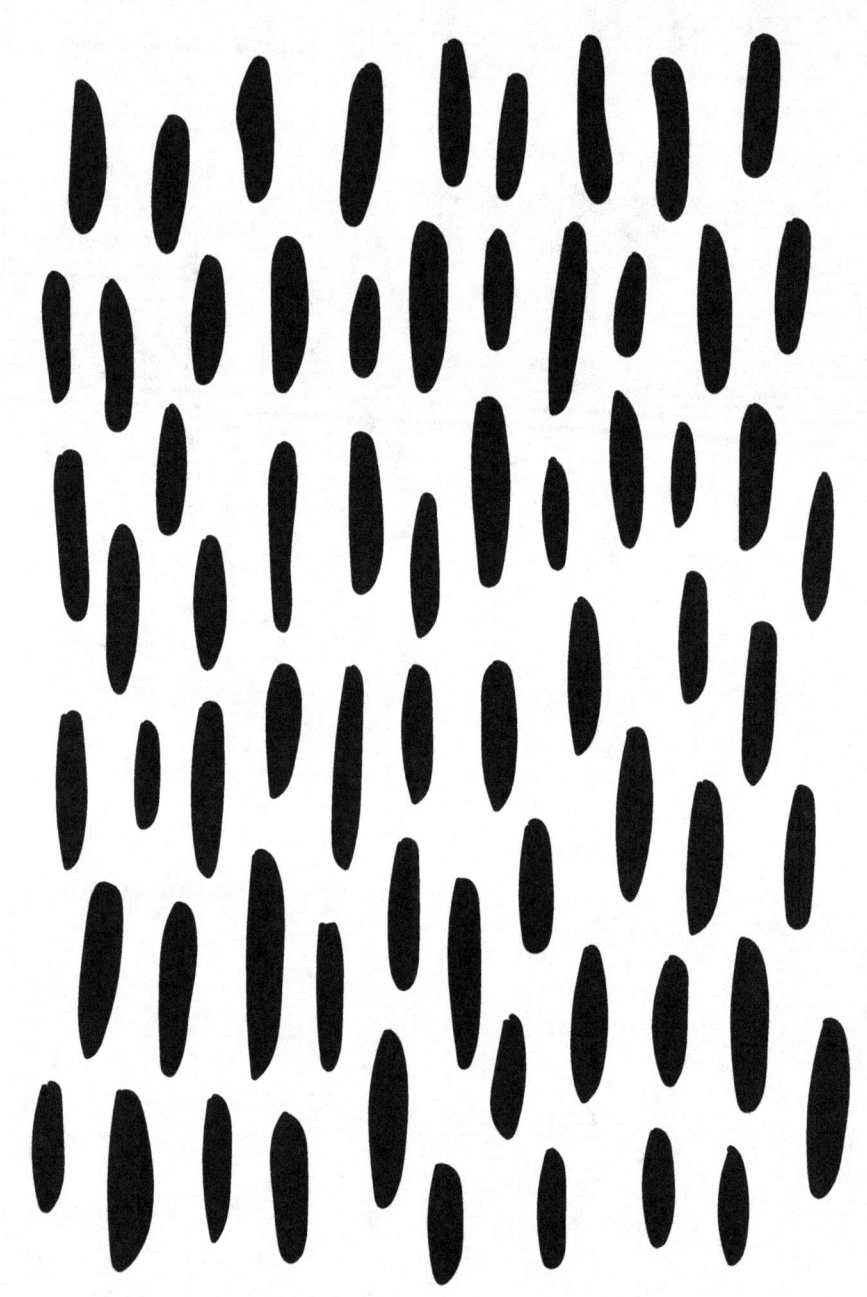

LEVEL 3

Find the right picture.

The children are playing soccer in the park.

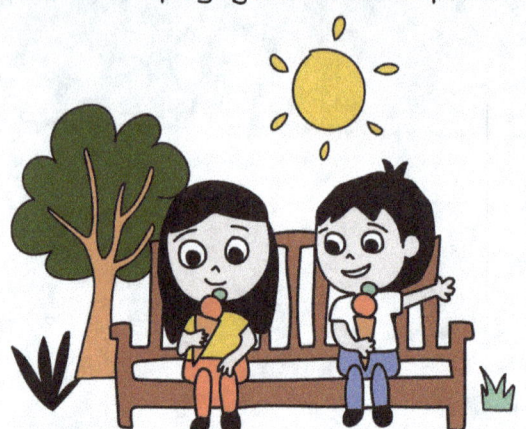

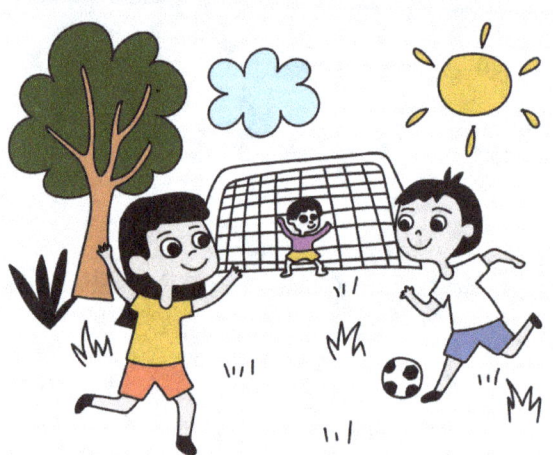

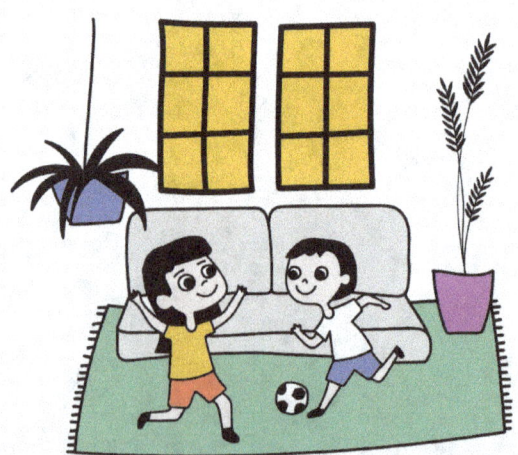

Find the right picture.

The girls are sitting on the floor, telling secrets.

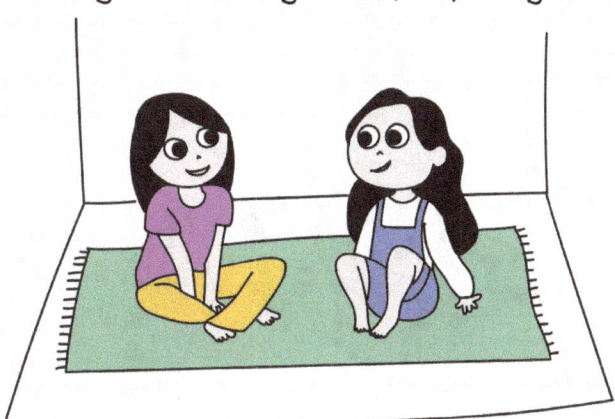

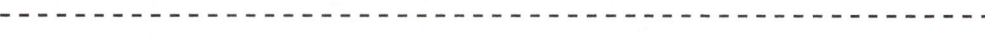

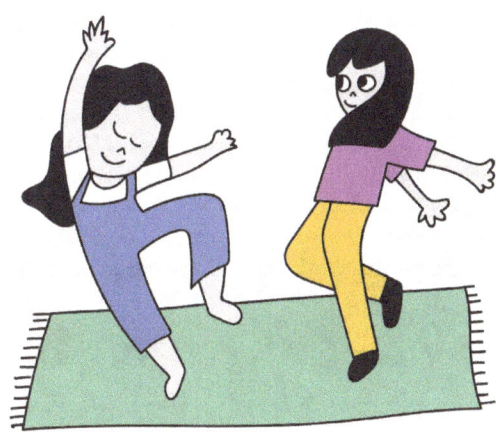

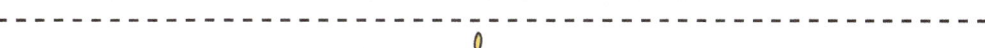

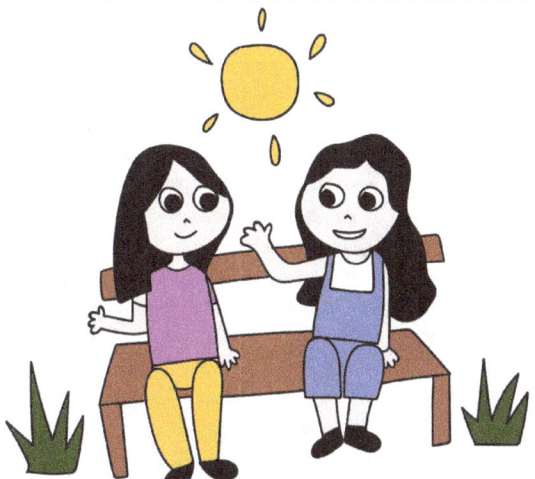

Find the right picture.

The children are in the classroom, divided into groups.

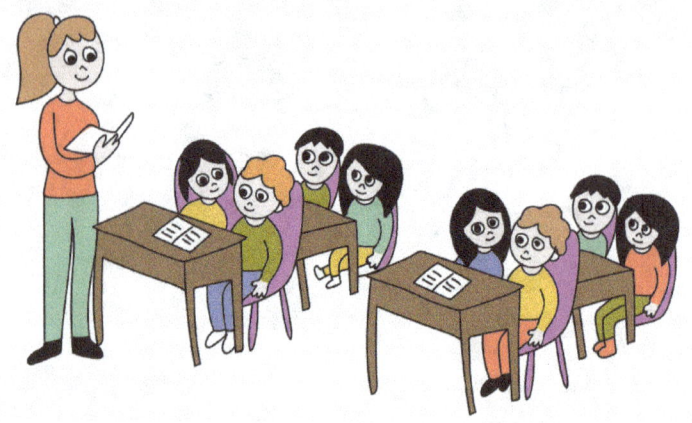

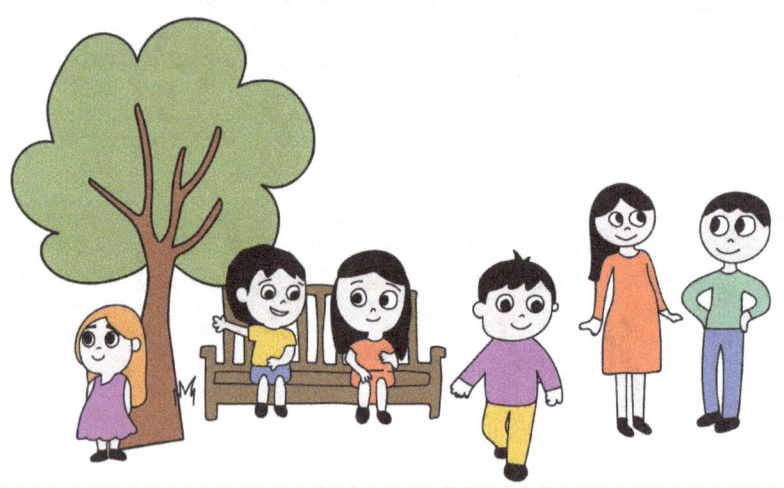

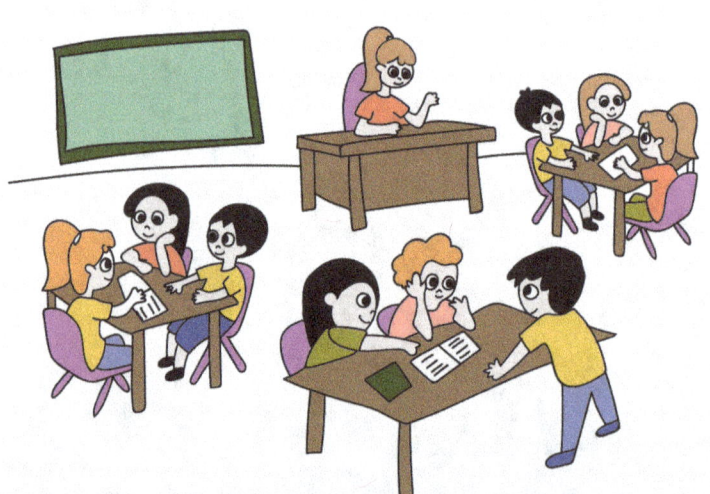

Find the right picture.

George is walking his dog in the park.

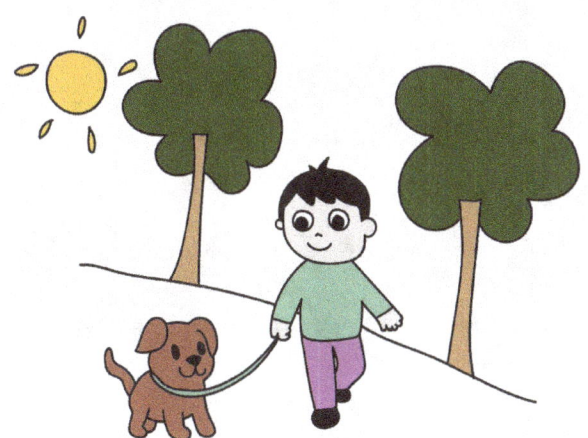

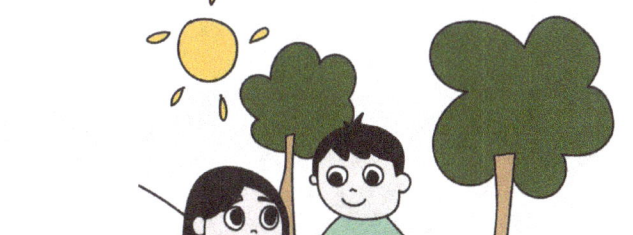

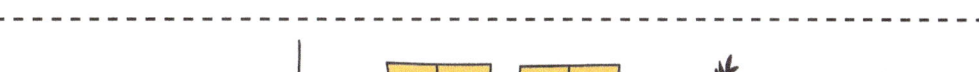

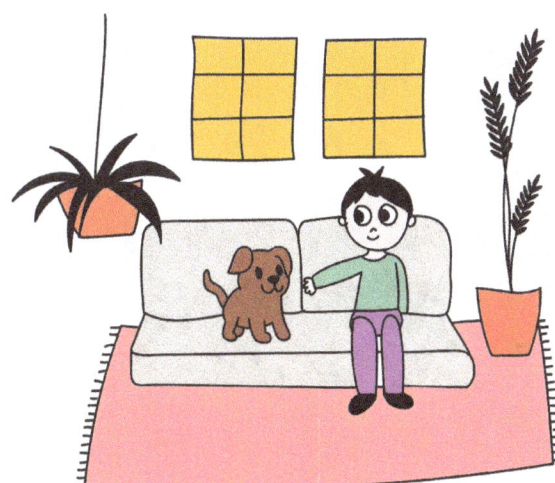

Find the right picture.

The dog is sleeping, and the cat is playing with the yarn.

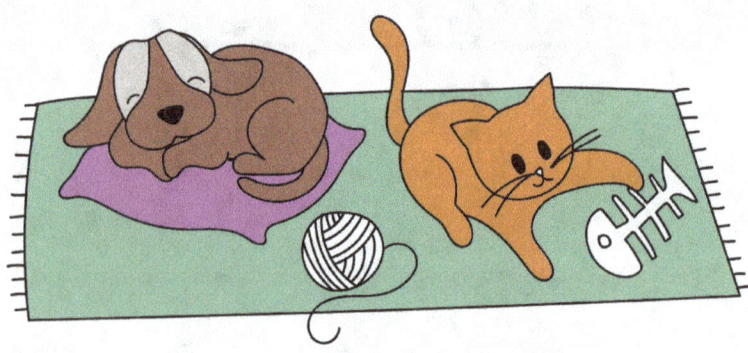

- -

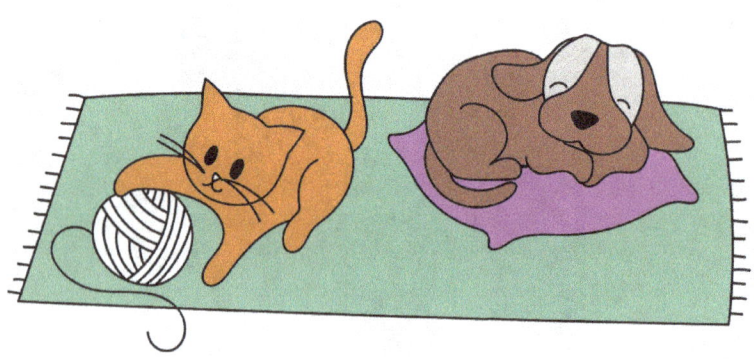

- -

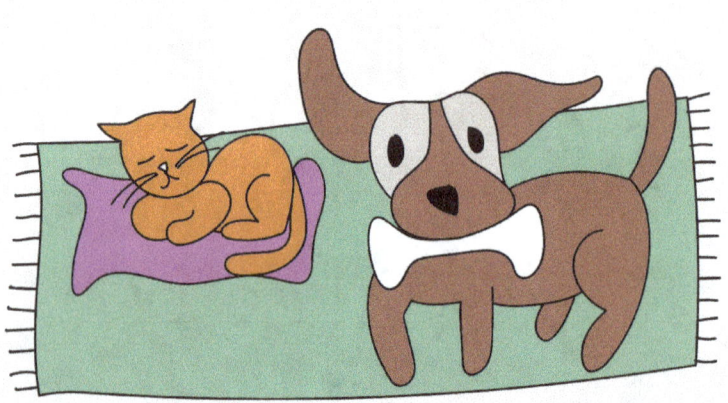

Find the right picture.

The children are building castles in the sand.

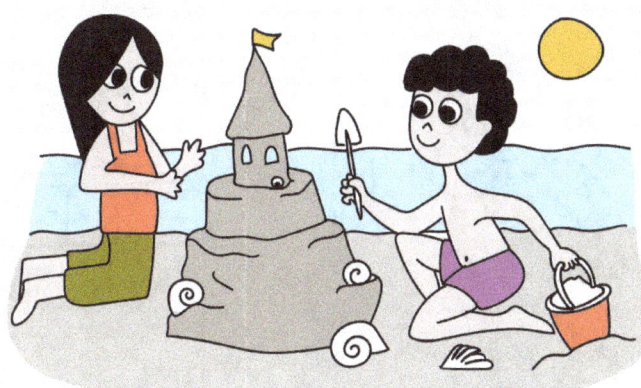

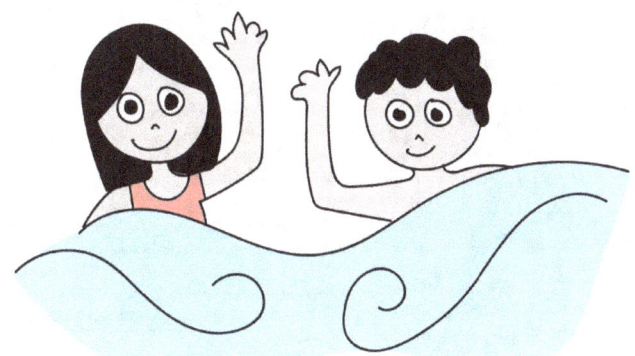

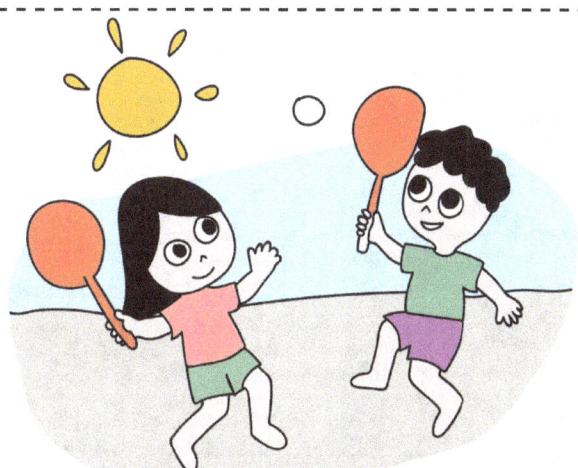

Find the right picture.

Mom is cooking, and Dad is watching TV.

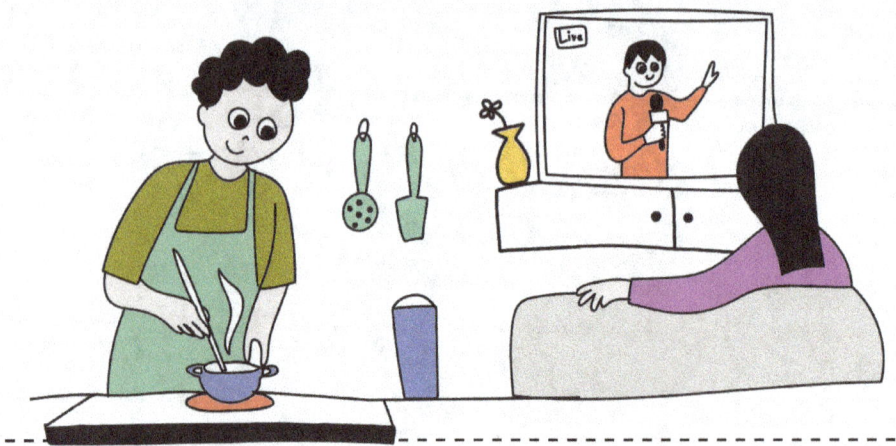

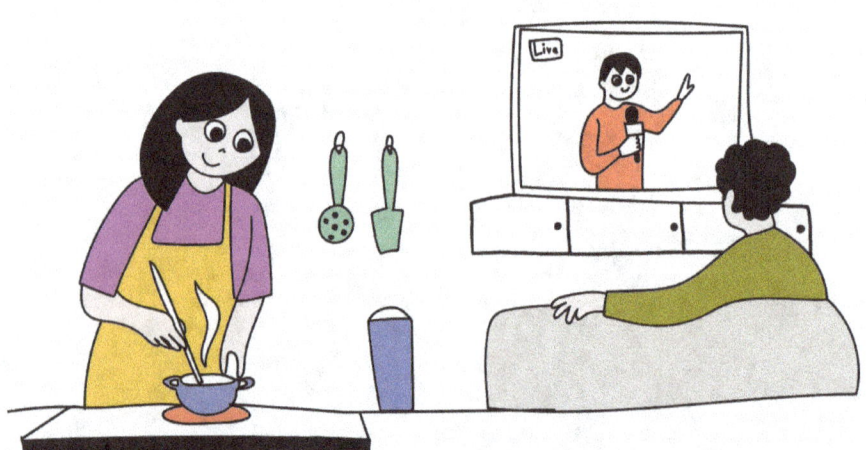

Find the right picture.

The children are traveling by train.

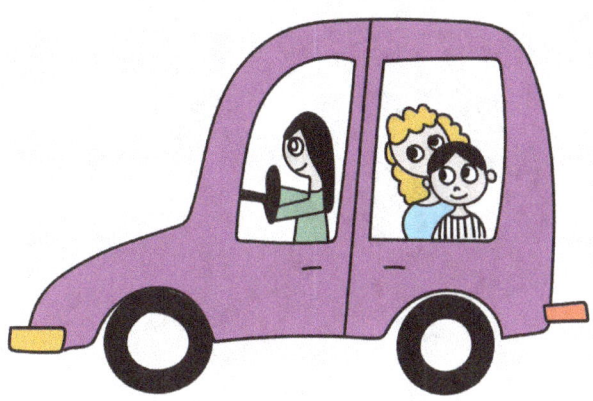

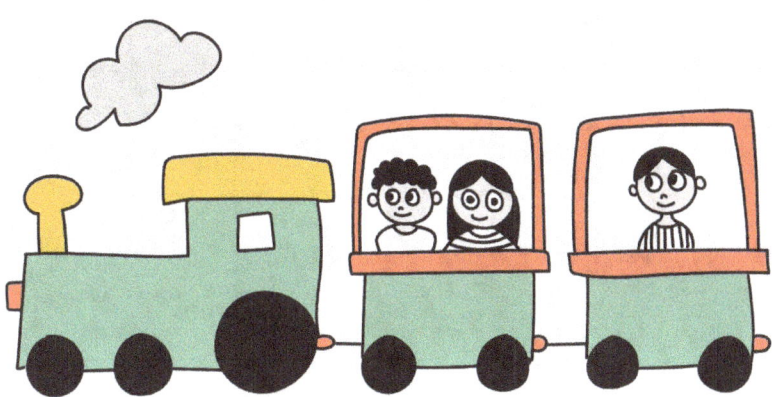

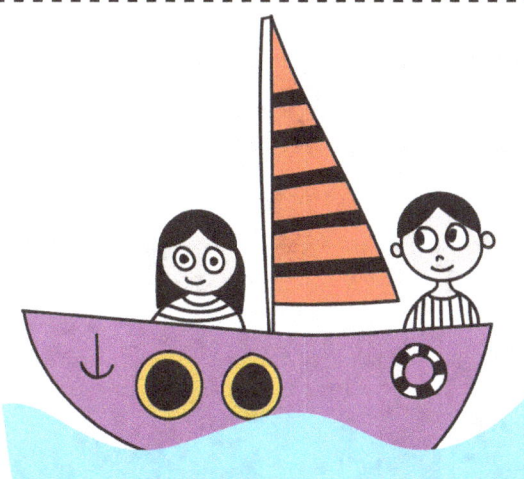

Find the right picture.

In the forest, there are different animals! Three squirrels climb up the tree. A fox is hiding behind a bush. Two clouds cover the sun.

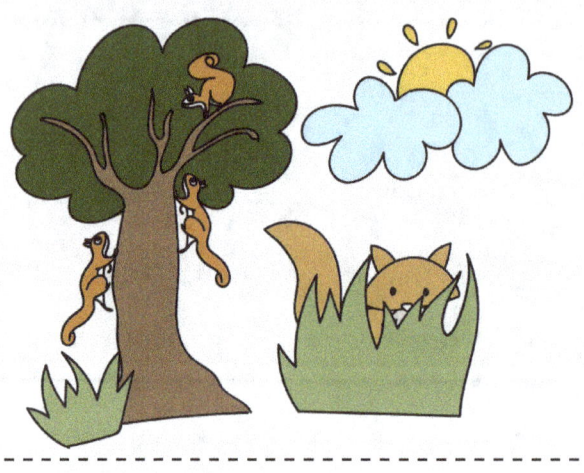

- -

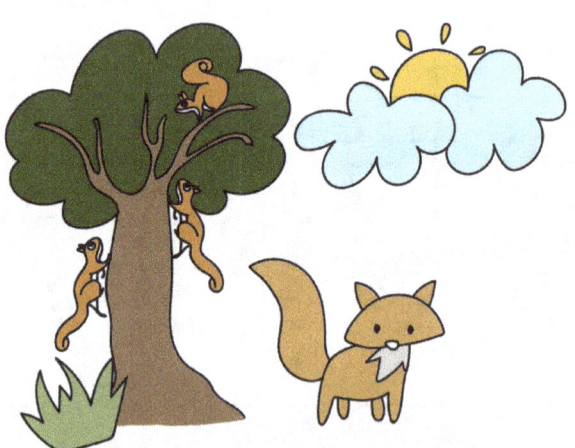

- -

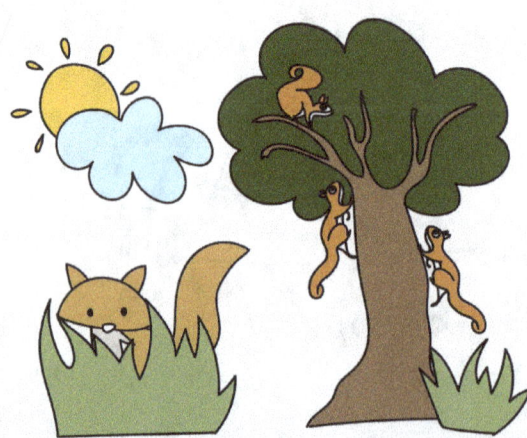

Find the right picture.

Grandma went to the grocery store and brought a basket full of fruit! She had three oranges, two lemons, four apples, a box of strawberries, and two peaches.

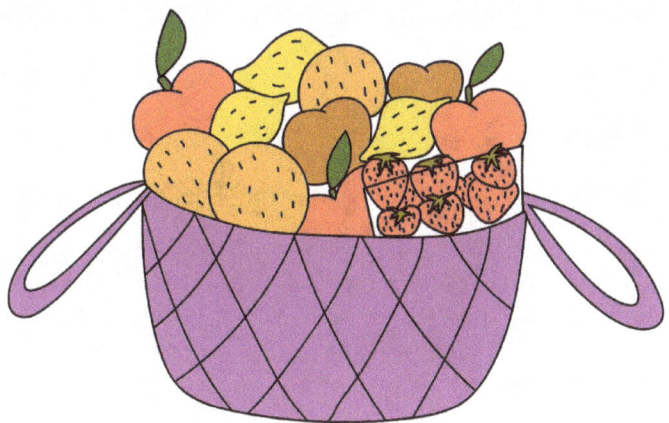

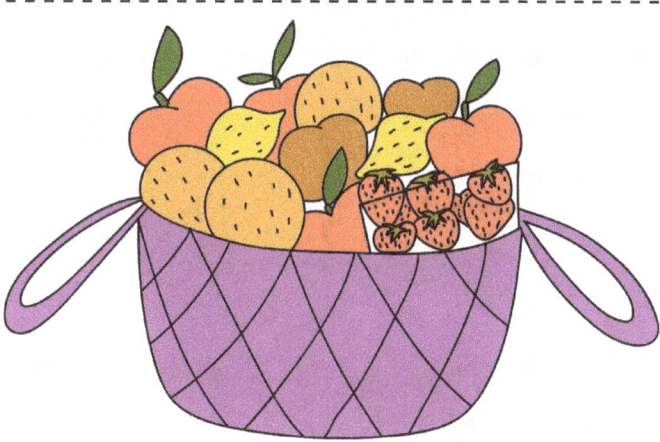

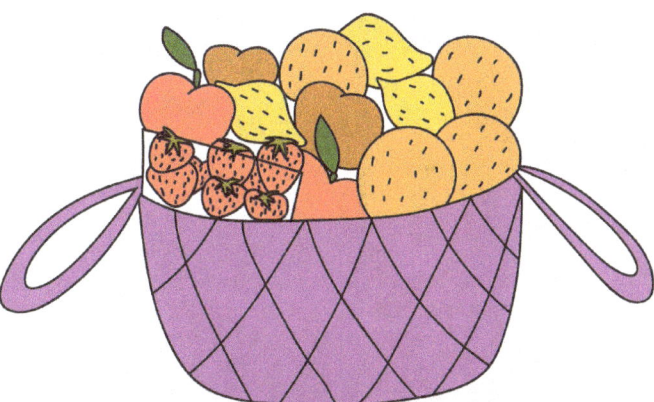

Find the right picture.

In the boat, there are four little animals: a giraffe, two kangaroos, and an elephant. Look! Two colorful parrots fly over the boat!

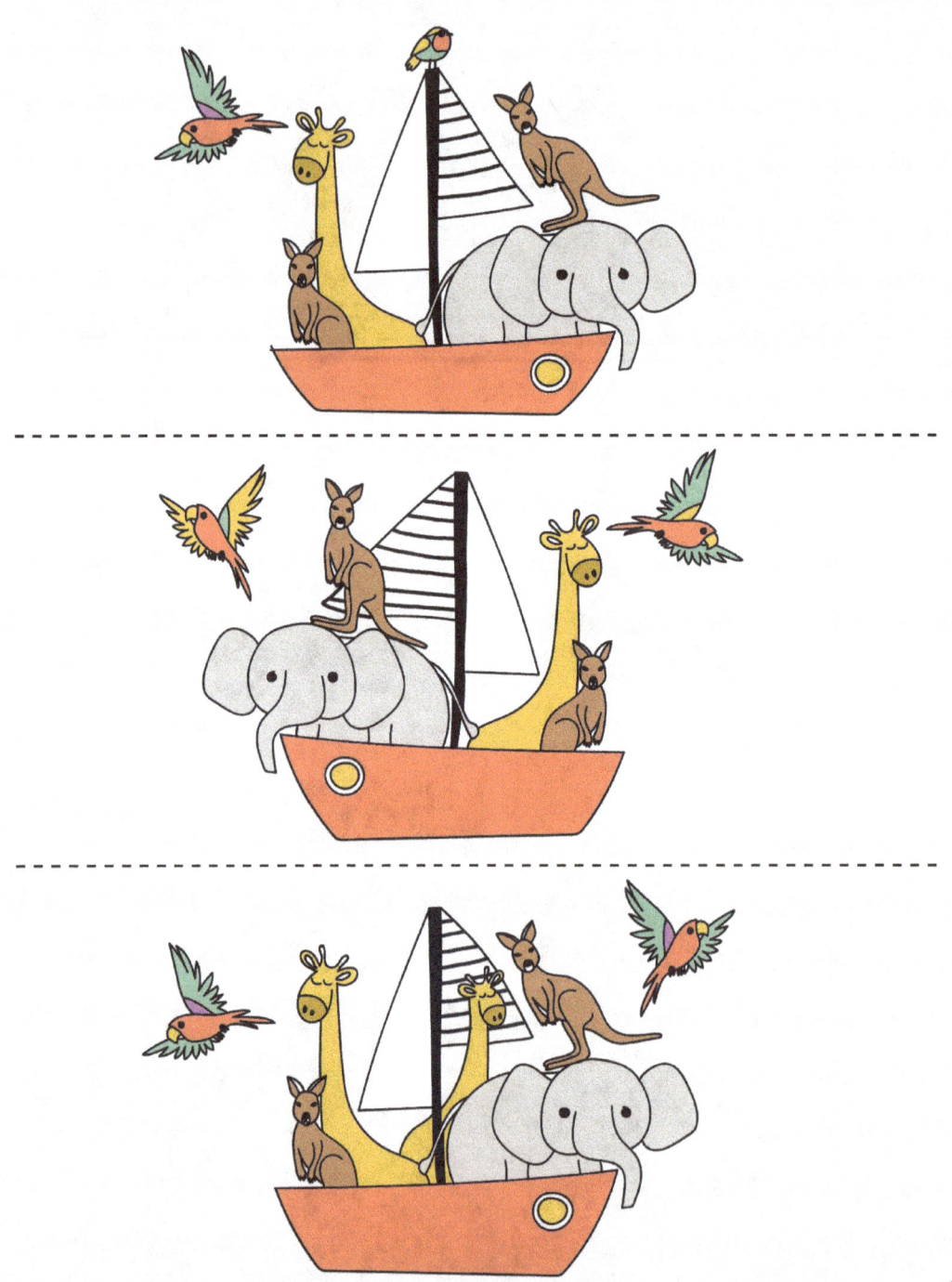

Find the right picture.

At the beach, my sister and I are building a sand castle. Mom is lying on the beach chair reading her book, and Dad is sleeping.

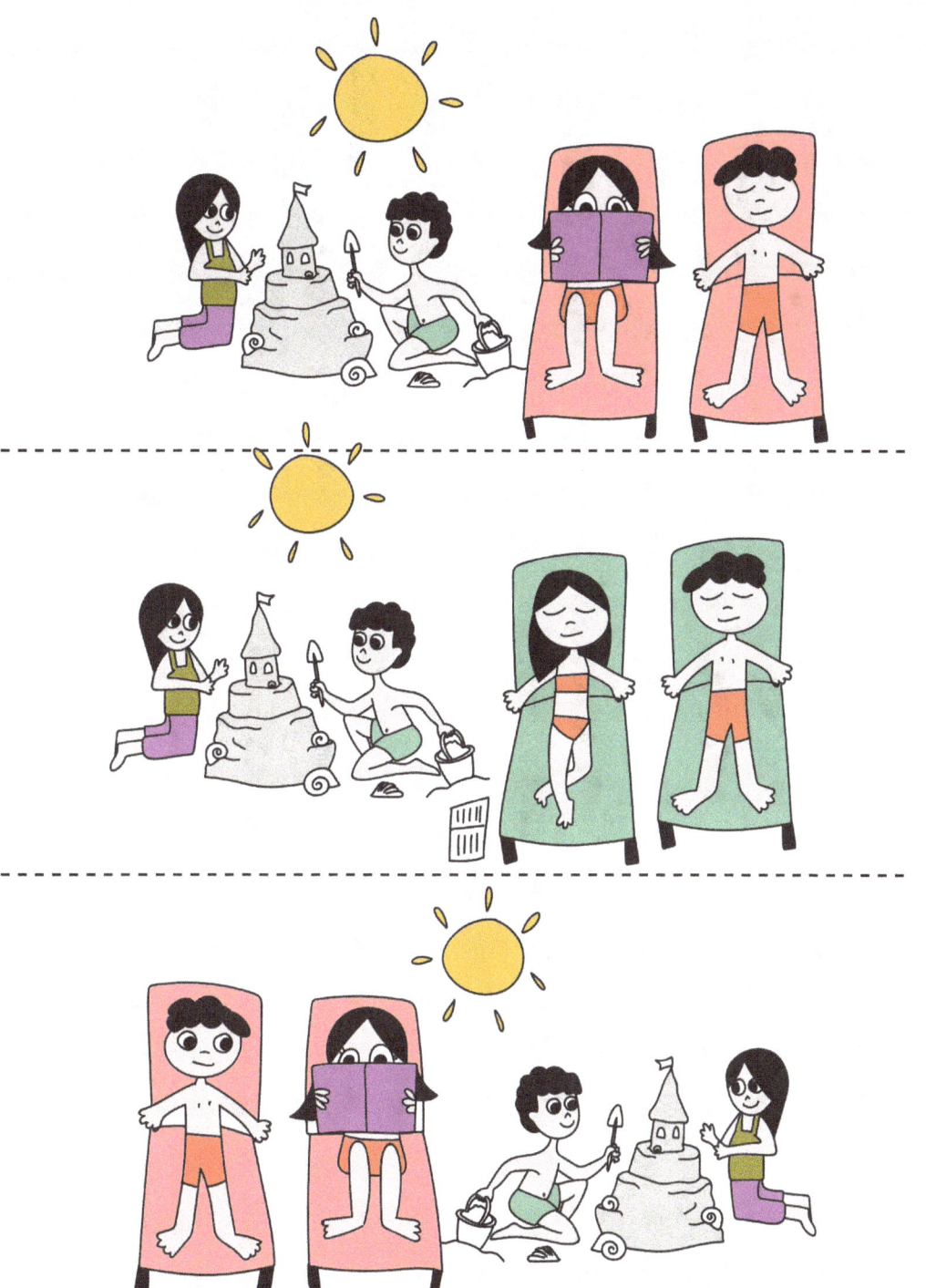

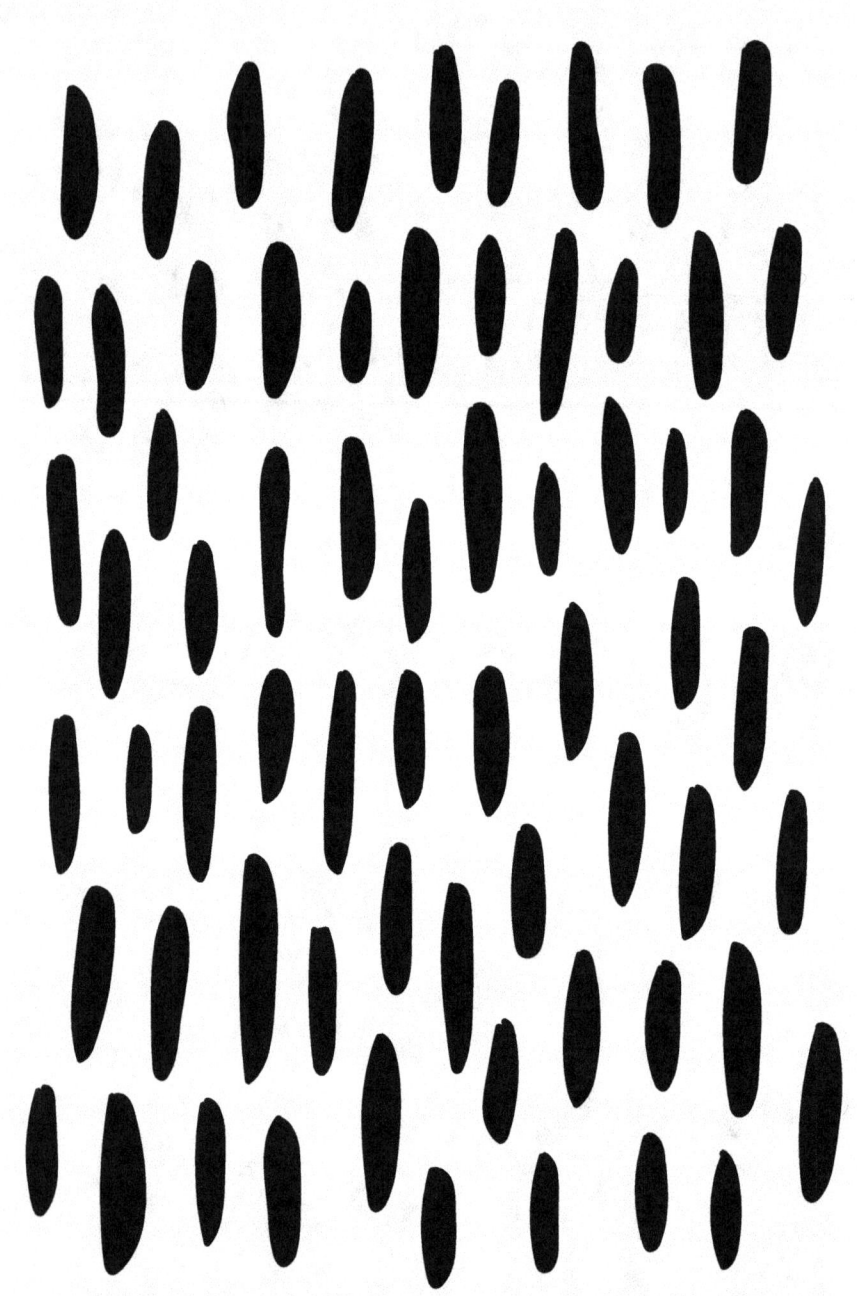

LEVEL 4

Read the text and follow the instructions.

Nick's garden

Nick planted roses in his garden. Every morning, he would wake up and water them with joy! After a few weeks, pink and red roses bloomed. He immediately cut them and offered them to his little sister!

1. Color the picture based on the text's information.

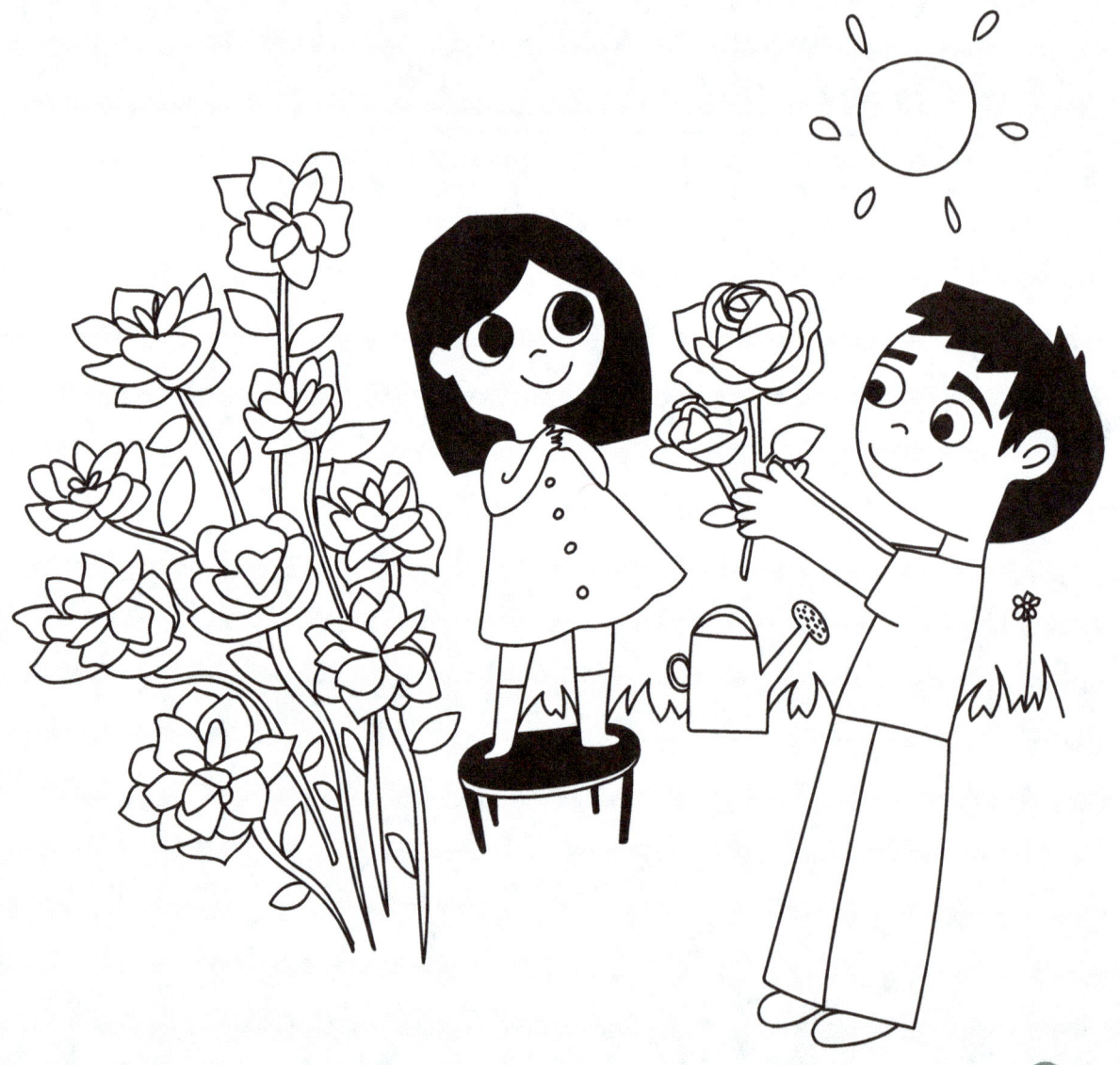

2. Circle the correct answer.

What did Nick plant?

A) Daisies
B) Trees
C) Roses
D) Violets

Where did Nick plant roses?

A) On the balcony
B) In the forest
C) In the garden
D) In the park

What were the colors of the roses when they bloomed?

A) Green and blue
B) Red and pink
C) Yellow and orange
D) Purple and white

Who did Nick give the roses to?

A) His mom
B) His sister
C) His grandmother
D) His friend

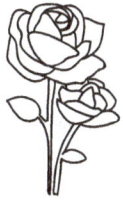

Read the text and follow the instructions.

My favorite toy

My favorite toy is a little train set my grandmother gave me for my birth-day. My little train is red with blue wagons. Some wagons are big, and some are small. I like to play with it every day after school. I imagine I travel to magical places. When it moves, it makes happy sounds, and its lights flash.

1. Color the picture based on the text's information.

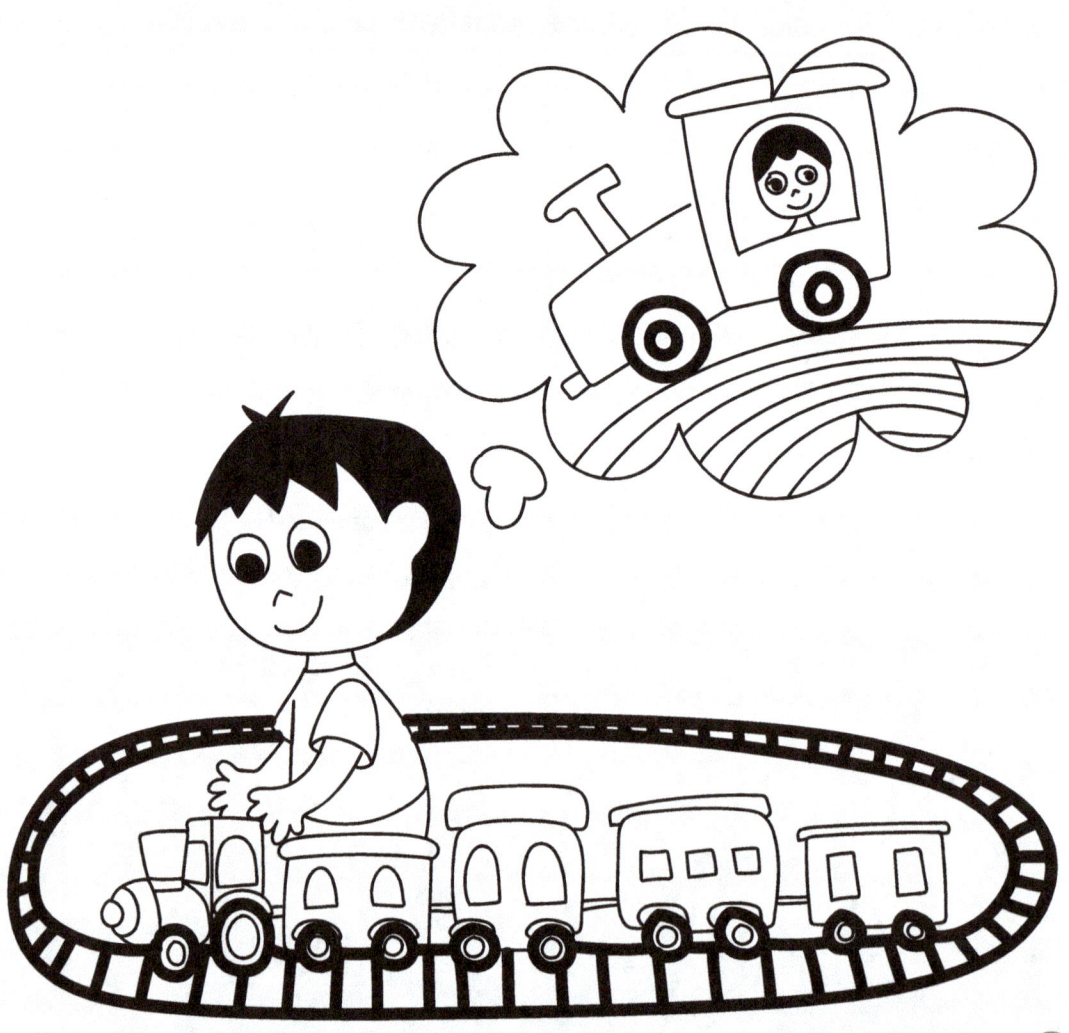

2. Circle the correct answer.

Who gave the train toy to the child?

A) His grandfather

B) His mother

C) His grandmother

D) His father

What color are the wagons of the train?

A) Blue

B) Yellow

C) Red

D) Green

What does the train do when it moves?

A) Goes very fast

B) Makes happy sounds and flashes lights

C) Turns off the lights

D) Plays music

What places does the child imagine traveling to when playing with the train?

A) Mountains and forests

B) Magical places

C) The sea

D) In the city

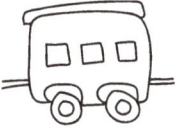

Read the text and follow the instructions.

Cloud

Layla has a small kitten with white and grey spots. She named him "Cloud" because his fur resembles a fluffy cloud. Every morning, the kitten waits for Layla by the bedside to wake up and play together. In her free time, Layla makes various fabric balls for Cloud to play with.

1. Draw a picture that's related to the text.

2. Circle the correct answer.

What's the name of Layla's kitten?

A) Flower
B) Cloud
C) Moon
D) Star

Why did she name the kitten "Cloud"?

A) Because he eats a lot
B) Because he has blue eyes
C) Because his fur looks like a cloud
D) Because he sleeps in the garden

Where does the kitten wait for Layla every morning?

A) On the couch
B) At the window
C) By the bed
D) Under the table

What does Laya make for the kitten in her spare time?

A) Food
B) Photo collage
C) Bracelets
D) Fabric toys

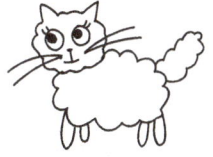

Read the text and follow the instructions.

The first raindrops

Mary was walking to school when the first raindrops began to fall. She looked up and saw the clouds covering the whole sky. She took the small umbrella out of her bag and happily went on her way. She loved the sound of the rain on the ground. Fall had finally arrived!

1. Draw a picture that's related to the text.

2. Circle the correct answer.

Mary was walking:

A) To the park

B) To school

C) Shopping

D) To her friends

How did Mary react when the rain started?

A) She ran to hide

B) She looked at the sky

C) She started to cry

D) She called her mother

What did Mary do when it started to rain?

A) Took her umbrella

B) Put on her raincoat

C) Stopped and waited

D) Ran back home

How did Mary feel when it started to rain?

A) Sadness

B) Fear

C) Joy

D) Disappointment

Read the text and follow the instructions.

Nick and his dog

Nick took his dog, Buddy, to the park. There, they played with the ball and met other children. Buddy really likes to run and jump. But his favorite game is when the kids throw him a stick, and he runs to catch and bring it to them. When it was time for them to leave, Nick whistled, and Buddy immediately ran alongside him, ready to follow.

1. Draw a picture that's related to the text.

2. Circle the correct answer.

Where did Nick go with his dog?

A) To the square
B) In the park
C) In the forest
D) To the zoo

What was the name of Nick's dog?

A) Buddy
B) Rex
C) Zuzu
D) Tommy

What was the dog's favorite game?

A) Running
B) Playing with the ball
C) Jumping
D) Catching and returning a stick

In the park, they met:

A) Other dogs
B) Other children
C) A small kitten
D) A new friend

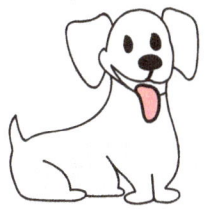

Read the text and follow the instructions.

The magic tree

In the middle of the forest was a tall tree with golden leaves. Luke heard this tree was magical, so he decided to explore it with his friends. When they arrived, they admired the tree's rose-yellow leaves that looked like gold and saw a colorful butterfly flying around it. The tree had small red fruits. They wasted no time and immediately tasted the fruits. They were the sweetest fruits they had ever eaten! All the children agreed that this tree was truly magical and made the most delicious fruits!

1. Color the picture based on the text's information.

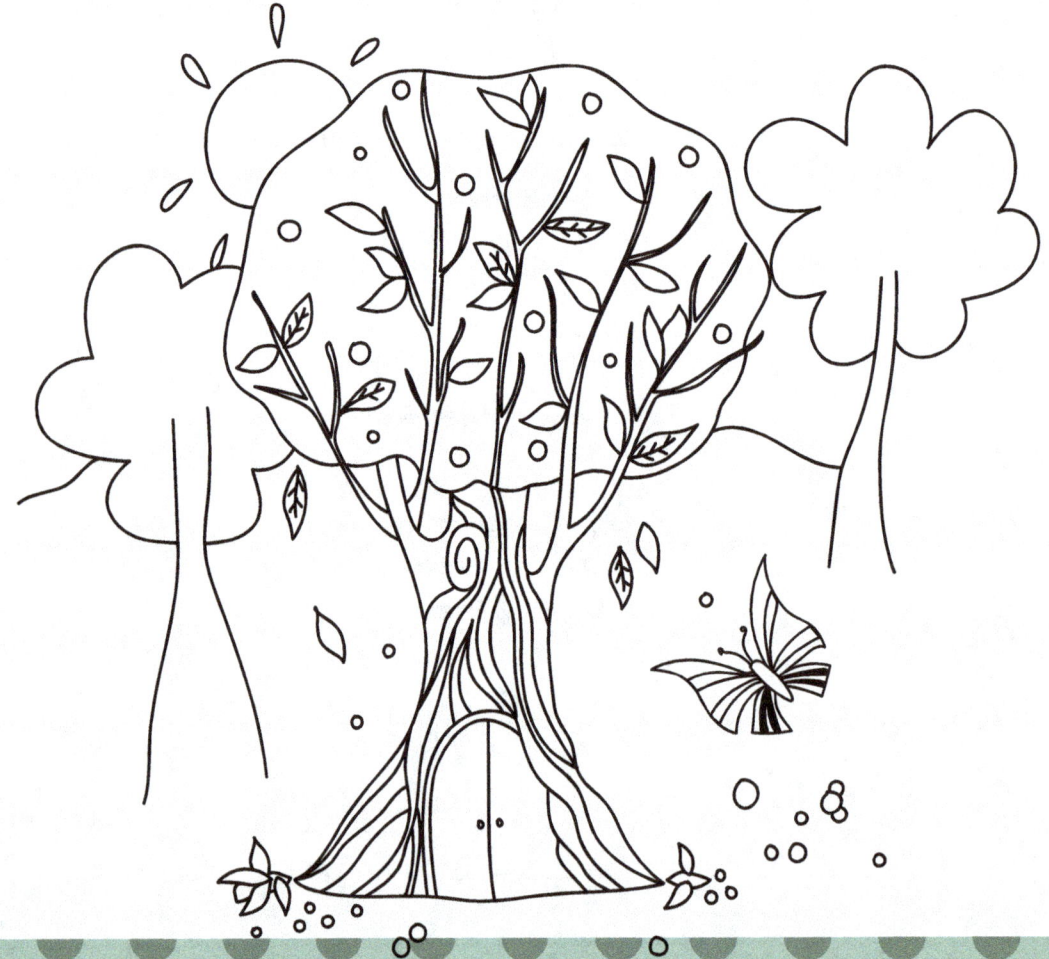

2. Circle the correct answer.

Where was the magic tree?

A) In the city
B) In the forest
C) In the mountain
D) In the park

What color were the leaves of the tree?

A) Red
B) Green
C) Golden
D) Blue

Which insect did Luke see on the tree?

A) A bee
B) A bug
C) A beetle
D) A butterfly

Why did the children think the tree was magical?

A) Because it had golden leaves
B) Because it was the tallest tree in the forest
C) Because it had the most delicious fruit
D) Because they had heard so

Read the text and follow the instructions.

My best friend

My best friend is Michael. We met in kindergarten, and we have been best friends ever since. We like the same soccer team, we like the same games, and we have the same favorite color and food!

Michael and I play soccer every day at school, and sometimes we get together on the weekends. We usually go to parks, playgrounds, even my house or Michael's. We like it better when we meet at our houses because we can play video games!

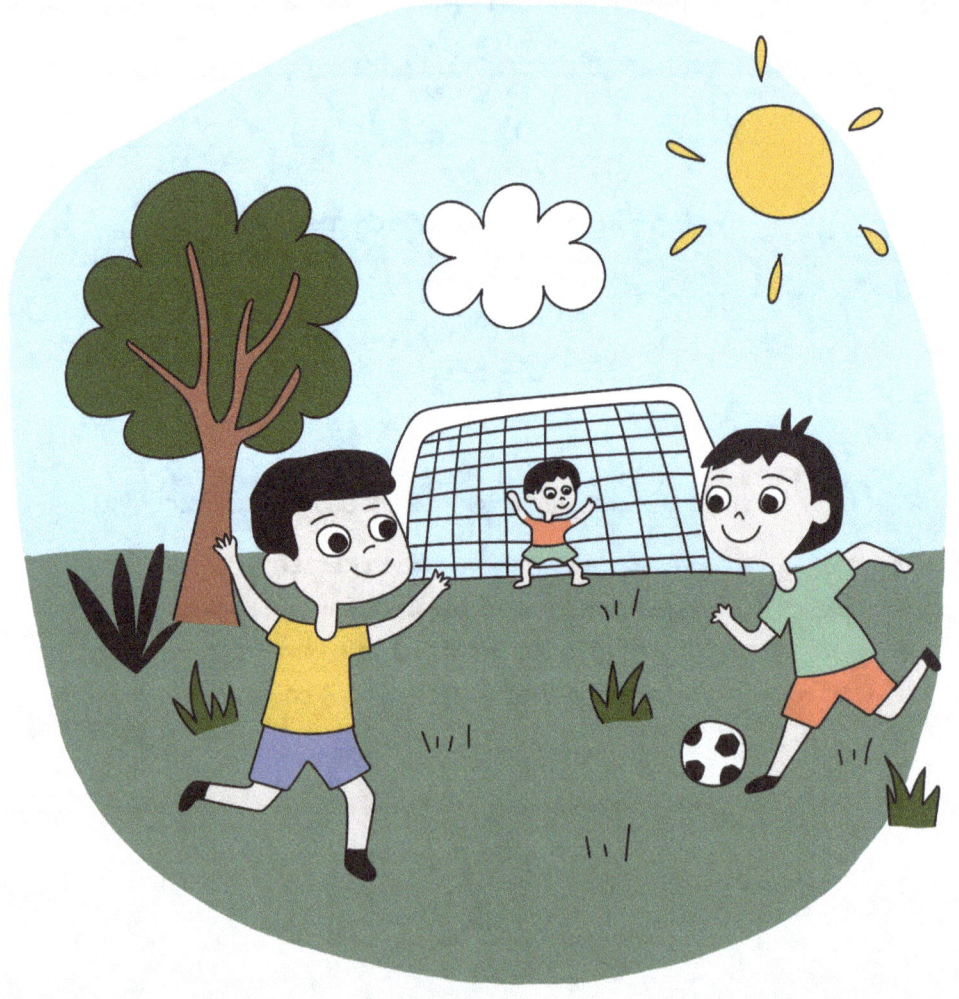

Circle the correct answer.

Where did the children first meet?

A) In the park

B) At the kindergarten

C) At elementary school

D) At home

What favorite things do both kids have in common?

A) Music and play

B) Soccer and food

C) Color and food

D) Food and music

What do the children play at school?

A) Soccer

B) Hide and seek

C) Basketball

D) They don't play together at school

Where do they like to be on weekends?

A) In the park

B) In the playground

C) At the mall

D) At home

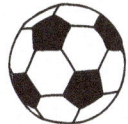

Read the text and follow the instructions.

Mom's birthday

Today is special for our family because it's Mom's birthday! We prepared a surprise party for her. Dad bought a beautiful bouquet of red roses, while my brother and I made a big card with our drawings. We invited grandma and grandpa, aunts, and a few friends. When she walked into the house and saw all the people gathered, the presents and the cake, her eyes filled with tears of joy. She hugged Dad first and then called me and my brother to help her blow out her candles together!

1. Draw a picture that's related to the text.

2. Circle the correct answer.

Why is today a special day?

A) It's Grandpa's birthday

B) It's Mom's birthday

C) It's Dad and Mom's wedding anniversary

D) It's my brother's birthday

What did Dad buy for Mom?

A) A book

B) A watch

C) A bouquet of roses

D) A piece of jewelry

Who made a handmade gift?

A) Dad and Grandma

B) The two children

C) The grandparents

D) The aunt

How did Mom react when she saw the gifts?

A) She hugged Daddy

B) Laughed out loud

C) Danced in joy

D) Her eyes filled with tears of joy

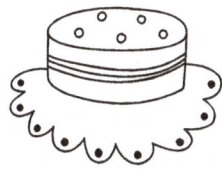

Read the text and follow the instructions.

Summer holidays in the village

Every summer, we visit Grandfather's village and have beautiful and carefree moments. The village is near the sea, has many trees and few inhabitants. Every morning, my brother and I go to the beach and make sand castles. In the afternoon, all the children gather in the village square, play games, and eat ice cream from the village café. In the evening, we sit in the courtyard and listen to Grandpa's stories about his childhood.

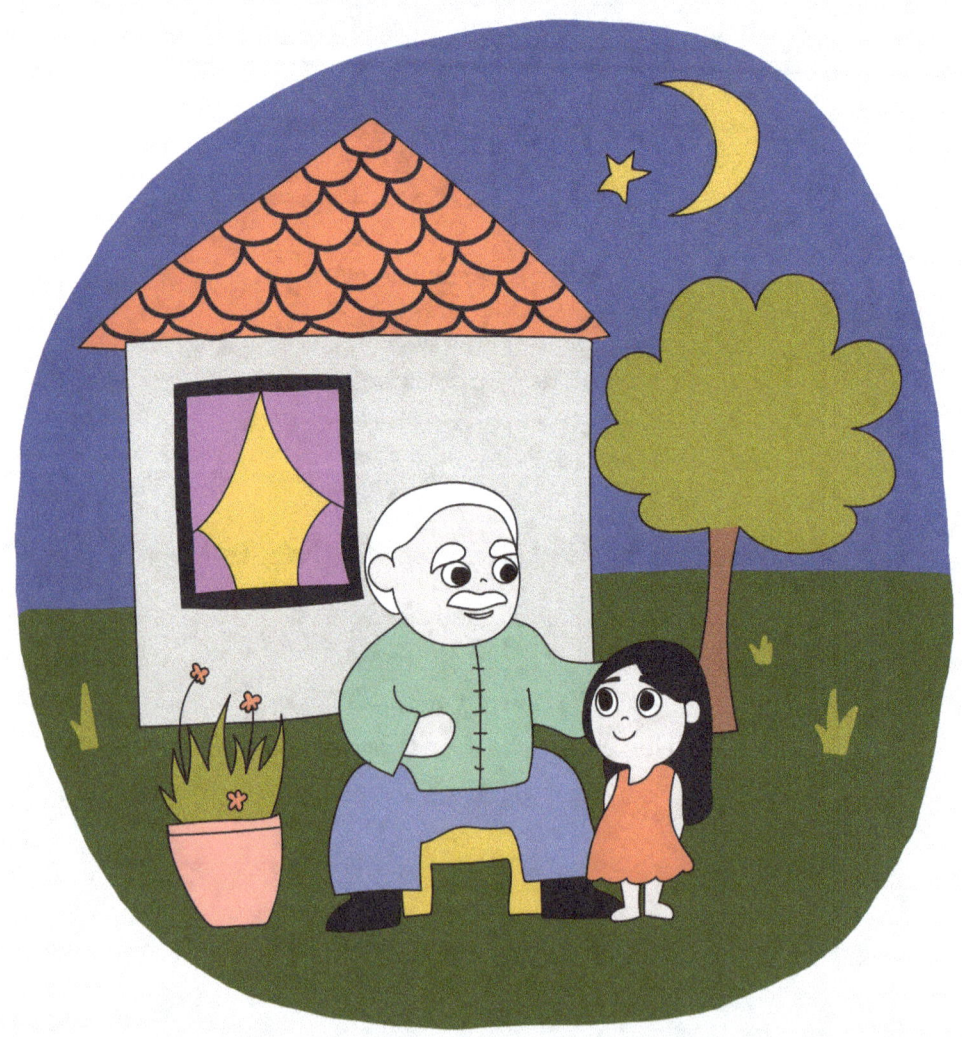

Circle the correct answer.

Where do they go on holiday in the summer?

A) To the mountain

B) To Grandfather's village

C) To Grandma's village

D) In the city

What are they doing in the morning?

A) Read books

B) Go shopping

C) Build sand castles

D) Play video games

Where do they play in the afternoon?

A) In the house's yard

B) On the beach

C) In the woods

D) In the village square

Who tells them stories at night?

A) Their father

B) Their grandfather

C) Their grandmother

D) Their mom

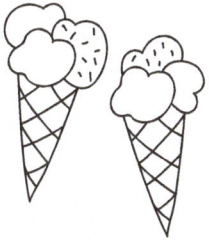

Read the text and follow the instructions.

On the island with my family

Every summer, I look forward to our holidays on the island. As soon as we arrive, the first thing we do is go swimming. The sea is so cool and clean! I love playing beach tennis with my sister. She always lets me win, and she thinks I have no idea! In the afternoon, we walk around the narrow alleys and buy little souvenirs from the shops on the island. In the evening, we go to dinner at small local restaurants and eat fresh fish.

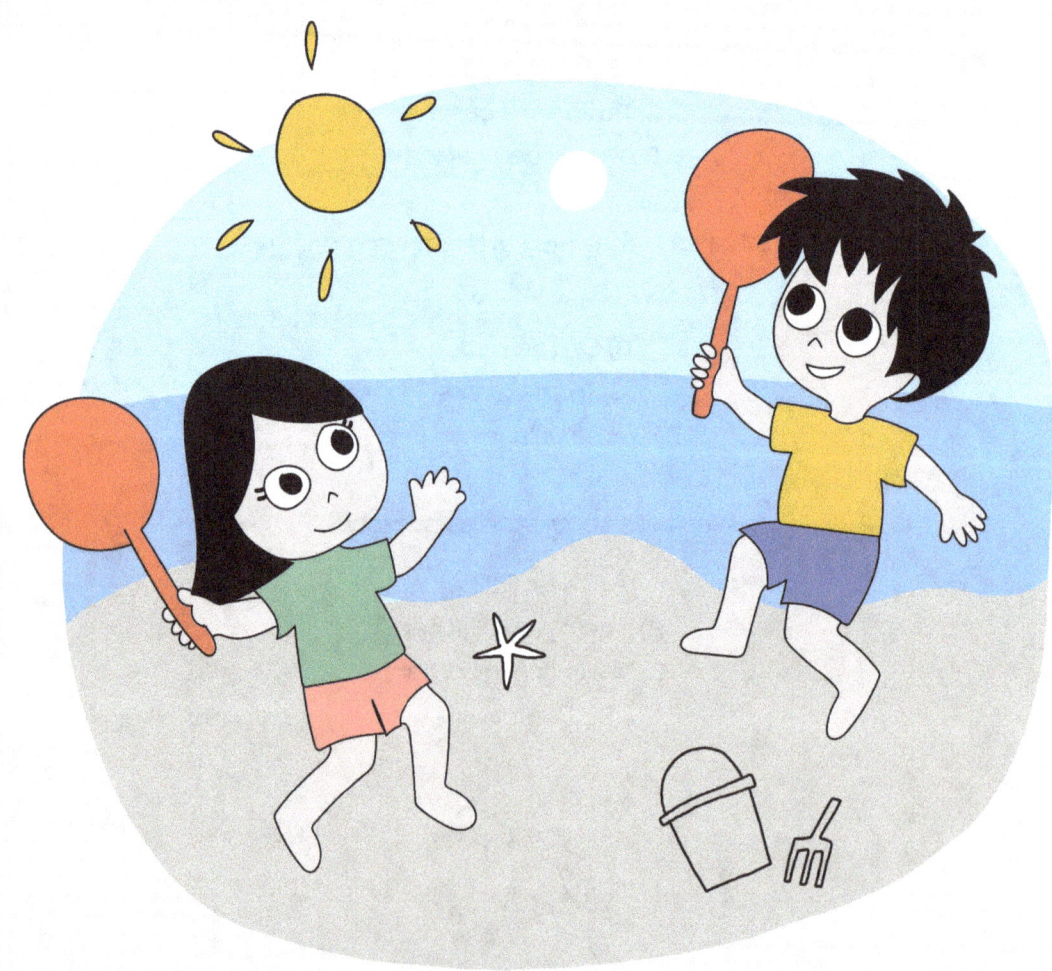

Circle the correct answer.

Where do they go for holidays every summer?

A) To the mountain

B) To the village

C) To the island

D) To the city

What's the kid playing with his sister on the beach?

A) Football

B) Beach tennis

C) Beach volleyball

D) Hide and seek

What do they buy in the afternoon?

A) Ice cream

B) Watermelons

C) Souvenirs

D) Clothes

What do they do in the evenings?

A) Watch the stars

B) Watch movies

C) Go for a walk in the island's alleys

D) Eat at local restaurants

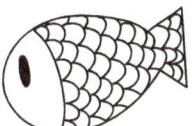

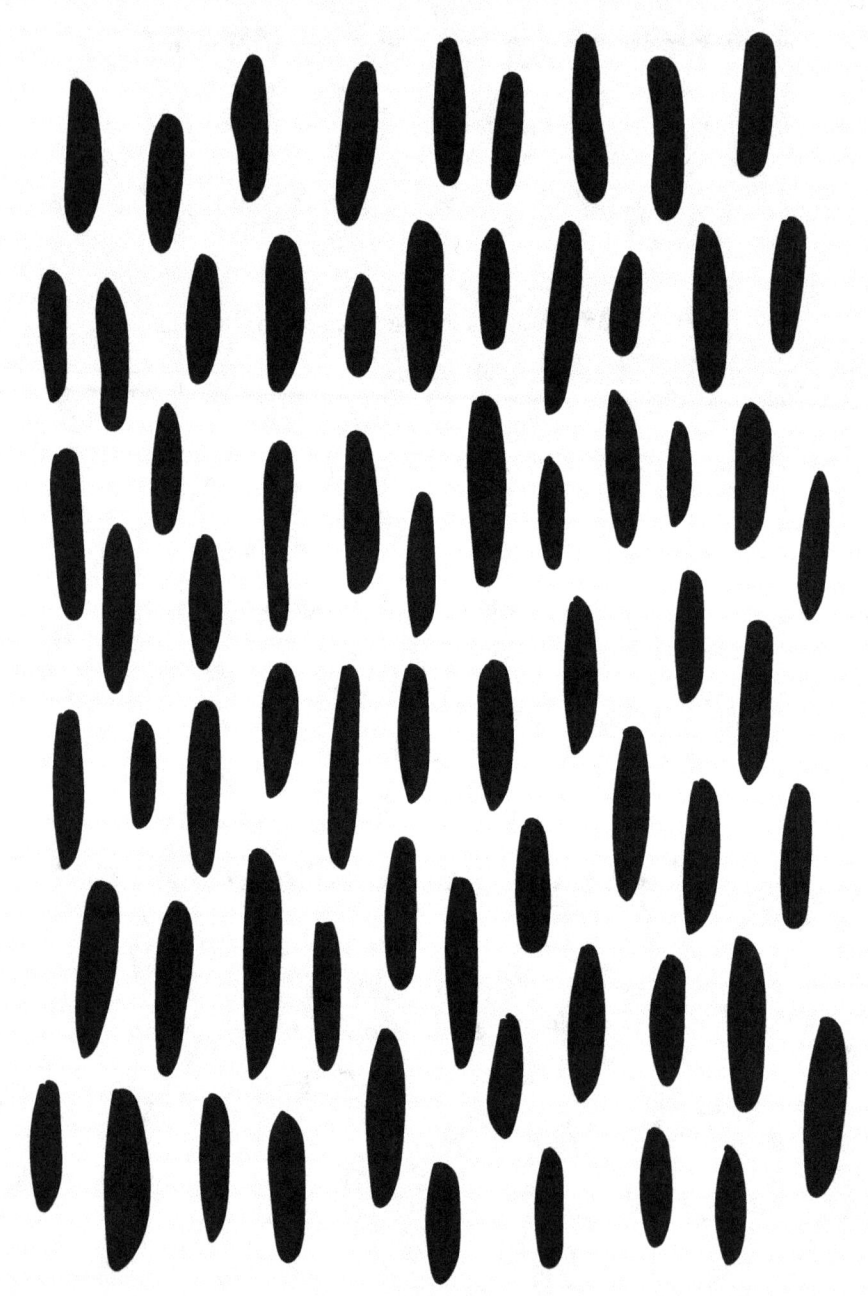

LEVEL 5

Read the texts and answer the questions in complete sentences.

At the zoo

Patricia and George went to the zoo yesterday with their mother. They saw many animals, but they liked the elephants, lions, and parrots the most. The funniest animal at the zoo was a monkey that made funny faces. They took pictures of it with their mother's cell phone. In the evening, they recounted their experience to their father.

Answer the questions in complete sentences.

1. Where did Patricia and George go?

_____

_____

2. Which animals did they like best?

_____

_____

3. Why was the monkey the funniest animal?

_____

_____

4. Have you ever been to a zoo? Which animal did you like most and why?

_____

_____

_____

_____

_____

5. Draw a picture that's related to the text.

Read the texts and answer the questions in complete sentences.

The invitation

Susan found an invitation in her mother's bag that read:

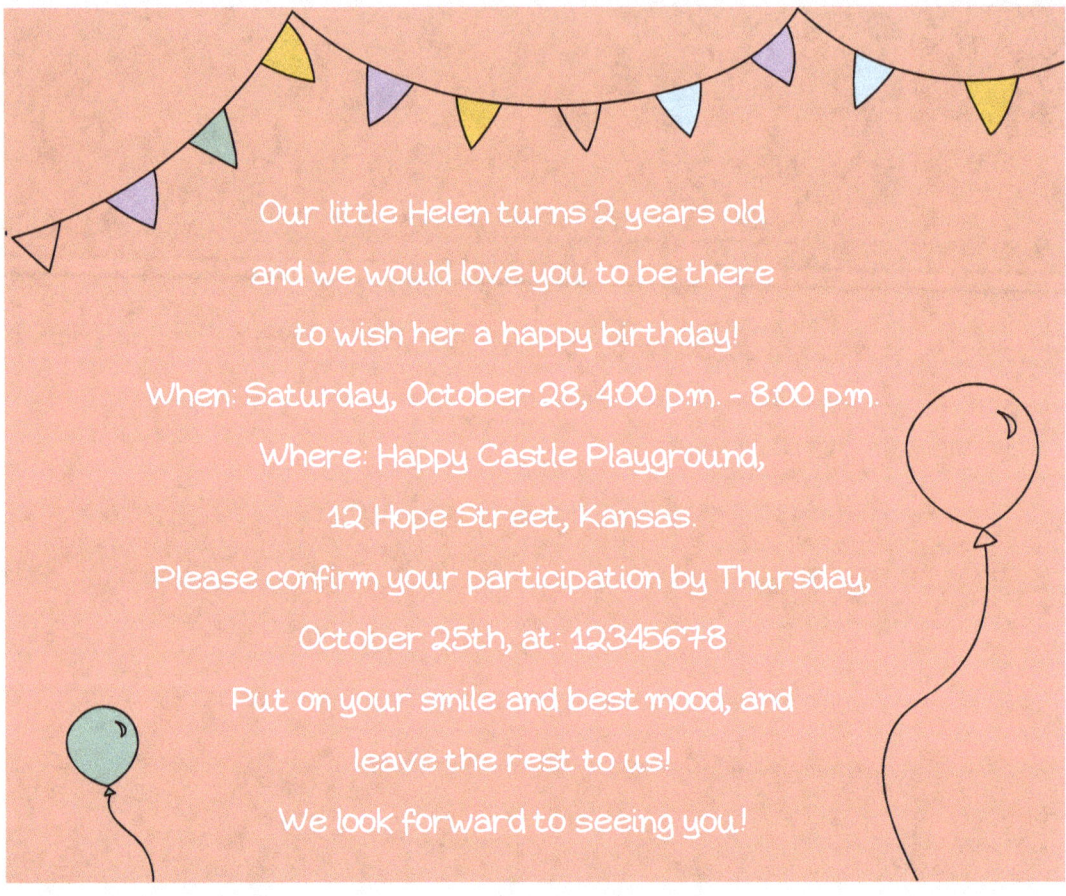

Our little Helen turns 2 years old

and we would love you to be there

to wish her a happy birthday!

When: Saturday, October 28, 4:00 p.m. - 8:00 p.m.

Where: Happy Castle Playground,

12 Hope Street, Kansas.

Please confirm your participation by Thursday,

October 25th, at: 12345678

Put on your smile and best mood, and

leave the rest to us!

We look forward to seeing you!

Susan's joy was indescribable! It was her little cousin's birthday, and now, she had to think about what gift to get her. "A teddy bear and a painting would definitely be nice for her," she thought and smiled!

Answer the questions in complete sentences.

1. Where did Susan get the invitation, and what kind of invitation was it?

_____

_____

2. When and where will the party take place?

_____

_____

3. What gift has Susan decided to give her cousin?

_____

_____

4. What gift would you give your cousin if it were their birthday and why?

_____

_____

_____

_____

_____

_____

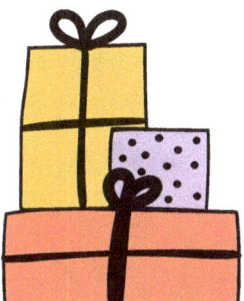

Read the texts and answer the questions in complete sentences.

My little brother

My brother's name is John, and he is two years younger than me! He has green eyes and brown hair. He is tall and a bit chubby.

In his spare time, he likes to play with his toy train, and we like playing video games together. At school, his favorite class is art because he wants to be a great painter when he grows up. Every night, he likes me to read him stories, although this year, he has also learned to read in first grade. Sometimes, Mom reads a story to both of us; that's my favorite moment.

Answer the questions in complete sentences.

1. What does John look like?

_____

_____

2. What does he like to play in his free time, and
   what does he want to be when he grows up?

_____

_____

3. What does John like to do every night?

_____

_____

4. Do you have a little brother or sister? If so, describe them!

_____

_____

_____

_____

_____

Read the texts and answer the questions in complete sentences.

My teacher

My teacher this year is Mrs Audrey, and I think she is the best teacher in our school. She makes class very fun and we play lots of games every day! Sometimes, she gets angry at the kids who make noise, but she tries not to yell because she says the rest of us shouldn't have to listen to yelling! She smiles every day, and if a moody kid comes to class, she always cheers them up! I am very lucky to have her as a teacher this year!

Answer the questions in complete sentences.

1. Why does the child think they have the best teacher in the school?

_____

_____

2. Why does the teacher try not to yell at children who make noise?

_____

_____

3. What does the teacher do when a child is in a bad mood?

_____

_____

4. Describe your teacher.

_____

_____

_____

_____

_____

Read the texts and answer the questions in complete sentences.

At the dentist

Yesterday, it was my first time at the dentist. The office was bright and full of colorful posters. Some posters talked about caring for our teeth, and others advertised products.

I sat in the chair and waited while the doctor sterilized his equipment. The dentist was polite and explained everything before doing it, and even when it hurt a little, it was good that he had already told me about it. When he was done, he gave me a small toothbrush and advised me to take care of my teeth.

Answer the questions in complete sentences.

1. What did the dental office look like?

_____

_____

2. What did the posters in the dental office look like and what was their content?

_____

_____

3. What did the doctor do while he waited for the child?

_____

_____

4. Why do you think the dentist explained every move he made to the child?

_____
_____
_____
_____
_____
_____

5. What did he give the child in the end?;

_____
_____

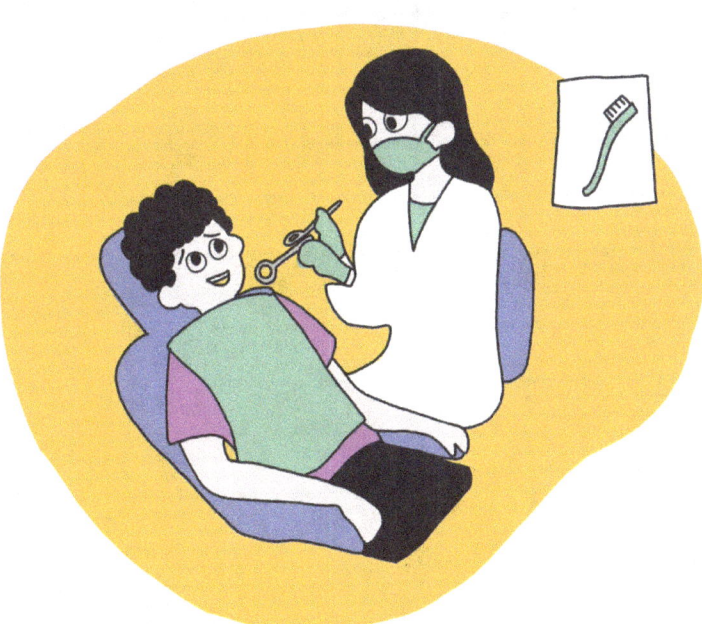

Read the texts and answer the questions in complete sentences.

The grocery list

Every time we need to go to the supermarket, my mom takes a pencil and a piece of paper and prepares a shopping list of what she will need. This way, she says, she doesn't forget the things she needs to buy because we're out of stock. She opens the cupboards one by one, then the fridge, and checks what we need. When I see her writing the list, I always remind her not to forget my favorite cereal and, of course, chocolates!

Answer the questions in complete sentences.

1. What does Mom do before she goes to the supermarket?

_____

_____

_____

2. How does she prepare her list?

_____

_____

_____

3. What does the child remind his mom to get from the supermarket?

_____

_____

_____

4. Prepare a short list of the groceries that your mom must buy.

Read the texts and answer the questions in complete sentences.

George's tooth

About a week ago, George's front tooth started to feel wiggly! It was his first tooth to fall out and he was really excited! But no matter how much he poked and wiggled it, the tooth wouldn't fall out. One day, while George was playing ball in the park with his friends, Daniel kicked the ball really hard and hit George in the face. He was scared when he felt something small and hard in his mouth. When he realized it was his tooth, he laughed and ran home to tell his mom and rinse his mouth. At night, he put his tooth under his pillow, and in the morning, the tooth fairy took it away and left a blue toothbrush in its place!

Answer the questions in complete sentences.

1. How did George's tooth finally fall out?

_____

_____

_____

2. What did George do when he realized his tooth fell out?

_____

_____

_____

3. What did George do with the tooth that fell out?

_____

_____

_____

4. Describe the moment your first tooth fell out.

_____

_____

_____

_____

_____

_____

_____

_____

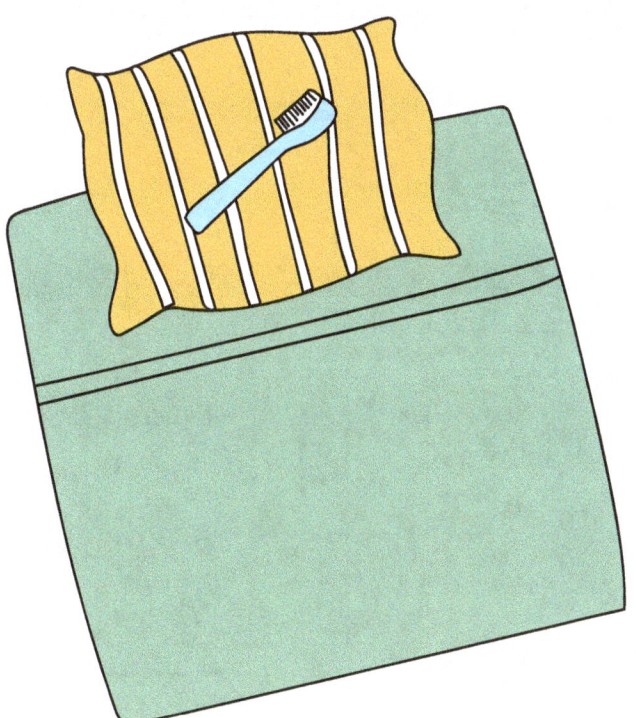

Read the texts and answer the questions in complete sentences.

The messages

1

We remind you of your doctor's appointment tomorrow at 8.15 am.

✓✓

2

Mom, I'm going to be late coming home. After school, I'm going to Nick's house to study together.

3

George, don't forget to pick up the kids from school.

4

Thank you for the markers you gave me. As soon as I finish my drawing I will give them back to you!

♡

==Answer the questions in complete sentences.==

1. Who do you think sent the first message and why?

_____
_____
_____
_____

2. Who do you think wrote the second message?
   Who is it addressed to and why?

_____
_____
_____
_____

3. Who do you think wrote the third message?
   Who is it addressed to and why?

_____
_____
_____
_____

4. Who do you think wrote the fourth message?
   Who is it addressed to and why?

_____
_____
_____
_____

Read the texts and answer the questions in complete sentences.

The birds of summer

The birds of summer are the swallows! Swallows are small birds with long, thin wings. They always choose to go to warm countries. Many say their return marks the beginning of the warm season. Swallows make their nests by sticking mud in the corners of buildings. In their nests, they put their eggs and raise their young. When autumn comes, they start their long journey to other warm places.

Answer the questions in complete sentences.

1. Which are the birds of summer, and what do they look like?

_____

_____

_____

2. What countries do they visit, and what does their arrival mean?

_____

_____

_____

3. Where do swallows build their nests and how?

_____

_____

_____

4. When do they leave one country and go to another?

_____

_____

_____

Read the texts and answer the questions in complete sentences.

Grandma's house

Grandma's house is in a small village in Texas. It's an old stone house with brown shutters. In her garden, orange and pomegranate trees bear fruit every year, and Grandma gives them to her children and grandchildren. In the house, there's a small kitchen where Grandma cooks food. On Sundays, the whole family gathers to eat. Every time we visit her, she greets us with a sweet smile, and she wishes us well when we leave.

Answer the questions in complete sentences.

1. Where is Grandma's house and what does it look like?

2. What trees does Grandma have in her garden, and what does she do with their fruit?

3. When do they visit Grandma?

4. How does Grandma welcome them and how does she say goodbye?

Read the texts and answer the questions in complete sentences.

Marina's garden

Marina has a small garden at the back of her house that is full of colors. Every morning, before school, she spends some time tending to her flowers and plants. She loves all the flowers in her garden, but a little more than the others she loves a pink rose that bloomed two days ago. Marina talks to it. She believes that flowers can understand her, so she shares her secrets with it. One morning, she sees a butterfly flying near the rose and smiles because she thinks her flower won't be lonely while she's at school!

Answer the questions in complete sentences.

1. Where is Marina's garden?

_____

_____

2. What does Marina do every morning before she goes to school?

_____

_____

3. What is Marina's favorite flower and what is its color?

_____

_____

4. How did Marina react when she saw the butterfly near the rose and why?

_____

_____

_____

_____

5. Draw a picture of Marina's garden.

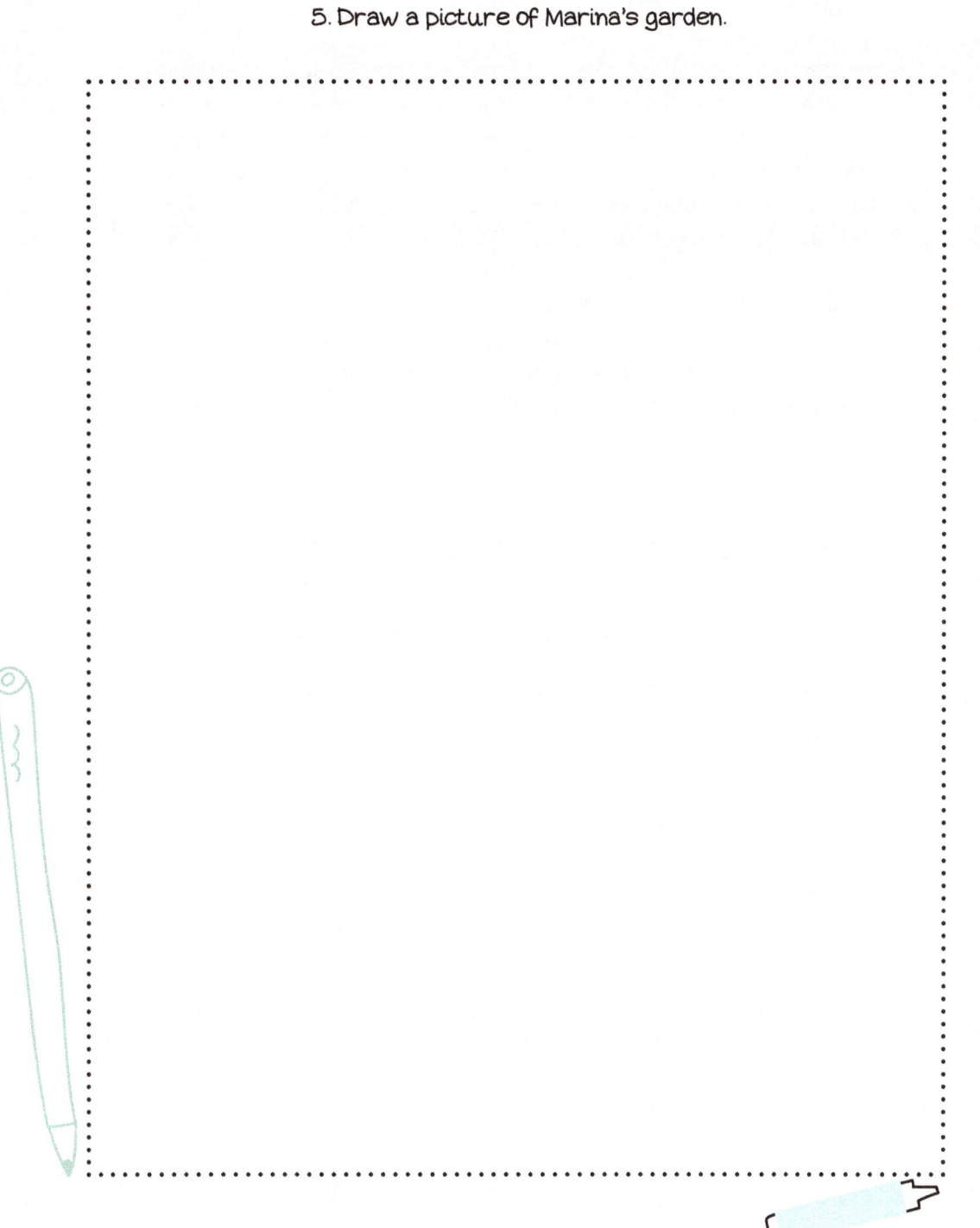

Read the texts and answer the questions in complete sentences.

At the museum

On Tuesday, our class went on a trip to our city's history museum. We set off early morning from school in a big yellow bus. We all wore the red hats we had been given to be easily identified. Our guide at the museum, Mr. Liam, showed us ancient artifacts such as coins and household utensils. He told us stories of the very old times, the value of coins in those days, and the use of many objects.

Many children were fascinated by the knights' armor and the weapons on display. During our visit, we took notes to use in our school project and some of us drew sketches. Before we left, our class took a photo together at the museum entrance. It was a great day, and we all learned a lot about our town's history.

Answer the questions in complete sentences.

1. When and where did the students go on a trip?

_____

_____

_____

2. Why did the children wear hats and what color were the hats?

_____

_____

_____

3. What objects did the children see in the museum
and why did they take notes?

_____

_____

_____

4. Where did the children take their photo before they left the museum and how do you think they spent their time?

_____

_____

_____

_____

_____

_____

5. Have you ever been to a museum? What did you like best?

_____

_____

_____

_____

_____

_____

_____

_____

_____

Read the texts and answer the questions in complete sentences.

Henry's accident

On a sunny day, Henry woke up early to get to school before the bell rang. He put on his new sneakers and left the house with his schoolbag full of books. As he walked past the old bakery in the neighborhood, the smell of freshly baked bread made him keep his eyes fixed on the bread pan visible from the window. Unfortunately for him, on his next step, Henry slipped on a banana peel that someone had thrown into the street.

As soon as he fell, his bag opened and all his belongings were scattered on the sidewalk. A red-haired woman passing by rushed to help him while two young children picked up the scattered books. The red-haired lady advised Henry to go to the pharmacy across the street, which had just opened. There, the pharmacist treated the scratch on Henry's arm, advising him to be more careful.

Answer the questions in complete sentences.

1. Where was Henry in a hurry to go?

_____

_____

_____

2. Why did Henry slip?

_____

_____

_____

3. Who helped Henry after his accident and how?

_____

_____

_____

4. Describe an accident you had.

_____
_____
_____
_____
_____
_____
_____
_____
_____
_____
_____
_____

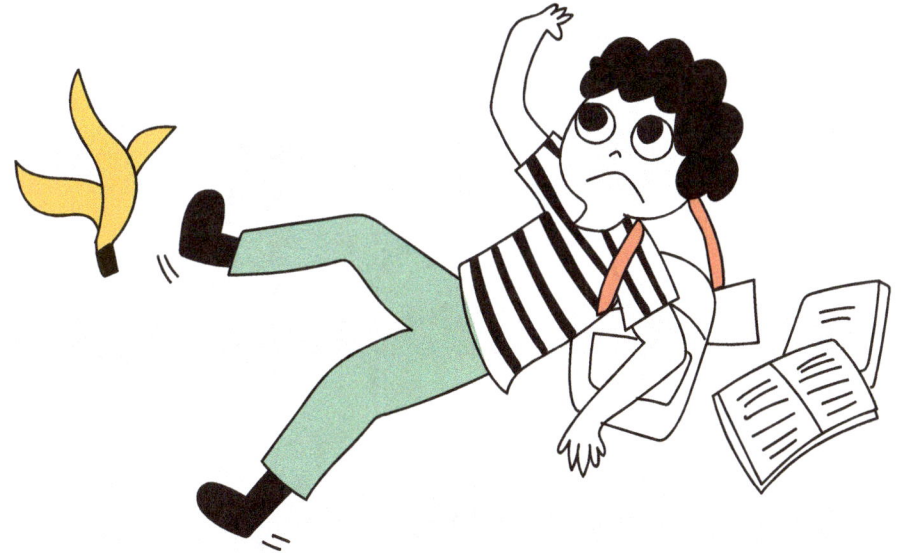

Read the texts and answer the questions in complete sentences.

Kate's birthday

On a spring day in April, Kate woke up in the morning more excited than ever! Her eighth birthday had arrived, and her day was going to be magical. She got out of bed and started getting ready for her party. In the garden, her mom had set up a table with a white and pink tablecloth, a large cake, and various strawberry and chocolate sweets, Kate's favorite flavors. Nearby, several gifts with colored wrappings were waiting for her.

Children from school, as well as relatives, began to arrive, bringing even more gifts and wishes. After playing tag in the garden, everyone gathered around Kate, singing, "Happy Birthday to you…" and watching her blow out her candles. After eating lots of food and sweets, the children continued their games. After several hours of play, the children slowly began to leave.

Late in the afternoon, Kate opened all the presents she had gotten. She was very excited about her new toys and the books she got. When she went to bed at night, she thought about her day, which was definitely one of the best of her life!

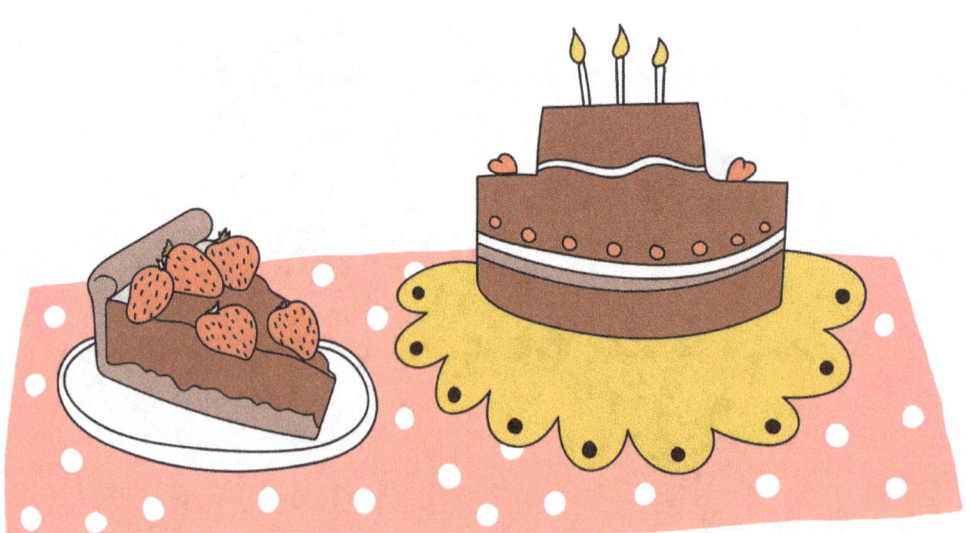

Answer the questions in complete sentences.

1. What month was Kate's birthday and how old was she?

_____

_____

_____

2. What color was the tablecloth at the table and
   what flavors of sweets were there?

_____

_____

_____

3. What game did the children play in the garden before the cake was cut?

_____

_____

_____

4. Did Kate have a good time on her birthday? How could you tell?

_____

_____

_____

_____

_____

Read the texts and answer the questions in complete sentences.

The camp

When Julia first heard about the "Lake of Dreams" camp, her mind was filled with images of woods, lakes, and tents under the stars. There was no way she would not go to this camp! As she packed her luggage, she chose to take the lantern her cousin had given her as a gift, her favorite pajamas with glow-in-the-dark stars, and a bag full of treats she hid in her room so her brother wouldn't find them.

Upon her arrival at the camp, the magnificent view of the lake left her speechless, as she had never seen such crystal-clear waters before. Soon, she met Chloe, a girl with red hair and lush freckles, and Brad, a dark-haired boy with glasses who knew all about the stars. The three became inseparable friends at camp, except at night when the girls had to go to the girls' dorm and Brad to the boys' dorm. Together, they shared unforgettable moments, such as morning swims in the lake and afternoon walks in the woods—all very beautiful memories for the children.

But their most exciting adventure was the treasure hunt, where Julia's group followed a map that led them to an old tree. Under the roots, they found a wooden box full of colored stones and chocolate coins, which they then shared with all the children in the camp.

On the last night, they had a big party by the fire, and Julia sang a song she had learned from her grandmother. When it was time to leave, Julia tried to hold back her tears. She made friendships there that will surely last a lifetime, making her very happy.

Answer the questions in complete sentences.

1. What is the name of the camp that Julia visited and what did she take with her to the camp?

_____

_____

_____

_____

2. Which two children did Julia meet at the camp? What do you know about them?

_____

_____

_____

_____

3. What did Julia and her group find under the old tree?

_____

_____

_____

_____

4. What did they do on their last night at camp?

_____

_____

_____

_____

5. How did Julia feel when it was time to leave? Why do you think?

_____

_____

_____

_____

Read the texts and answer the questions in complete sentences.

A different school event

On Friday morning, school seemed different from other days due to an unusual school event. The students were divided into groups. Each group would present to the parents and teachers a show that they had prepared on their own, without the help and guidance of a teacher. Early on, teachers and some parents helped decorate the event hall with ribbons and colorful balloons.

During a long recess, the children went to the courtyard and started rehearsals. Noah and Sophia practiced telling their story under the shade of a large plane tree. Next to them, another group of children were rehearsing their dance, and in the covered arena, five children from the choir were rehearsing their songs.

When it was time for the event to start, the parents filled the audience's seats. Cameras were ready to record every moment. Noah and Sophia's tale about friendship and cooperation won the applause.

Once they were done, the children of the second grade danced in cowboy costumes. The joy and enthusiasm made the school event memorable for everyone.

Answer the questions in complete sentences.

1. What school event was held on Friday? Why was it different?

_____

_____

_____

_____

2. Who decorated the event hall and how?

_____

_____

_____

_____

3. What did Noah and Sophia talk about?

_____

_____

_____

_____

4. Where did the dance team rehearse and where did the choir rehearse?

_____

_____

_____

_____

5. What did the second graders dance and how were they dressed?

_____

_____

_____

_____

6. If you had such an event at your school,
what would you like to present and why?

_____

_____

_____

_____

_____

Read the texts and answer the questions in complete sentences.

The new school

In her new school, Stella felt like a small fish in a huge ocean. At her previous school, everything was more familiar: a smaller building, familiar faces, and a courtyard where all the students played together. But now, most people walked past her without noticing her, and the yard seemed endless.

During recess, she sat on a bench near a large plane tree, watching the other children playing happily. A group of children was playing ball, another group of girls was drawing on the ground, and nearby, four boys were playing hopscotch on a court they drew on the ground. Then Magda, a girl with brown hair and green eyes approached Stella with a friendly smile and invited her to play with them. At first, Stella was very hesitant, but seeing Magda's friends calling her from afar, she couldn't resist!

The next few days went by faster than Stella expected. She became friends with Magda and many other children in her class. She started going to school with joy, looking forward to each new day. The "new" school quickly became "her" school!

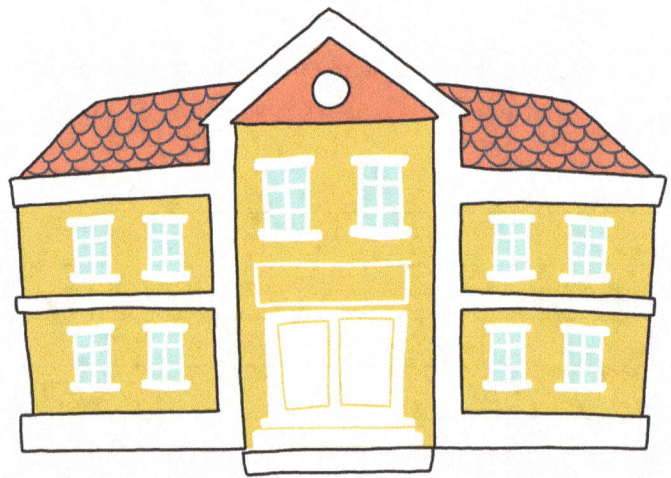

Answer the questions in complete sentences.

1. Compare Stella's old school with her new school.

_____

_____

_____

_____

2. What games were the children playing that Stella observed at recess?

_____

_____

_____

_____

3. Why do you think Stella was reluctant at first to follow Magda?

_____

_____

_____

_____

4. Do you think Stella liked the new school in the end or not?

_____

_____

_____

_____

Read the texts and answer the questions in complete sentences.

In the circus

It was a hot May day when Jonathan and his family decided to go to the circus, which had set up tents next to the city park. As they walked to the entrance, they heard children's laughter, music, and an elephant's trumpeting.

Once inside, a jolly clown with a red nose and big shoes greeted them, offering them a balloon. Jonathan chose a blue one, his favorite color. As they walked on, they saw the brave acrobats walking on a tightrope high in the air while the people below watched breathlessly.

At another point, a magician in shiny clothes made various animals disappear and brought them back, including a white owl and a kitten. Jonathan's favorite part, however, was the horse show, which danced in sync with the music under the stage lights.

When the show was over, Jonathan took a picture with the clown and bought a small acrobat toy. With a sweet smile and lots of memories, he wondered when he would have the chance to return to this magical place again.

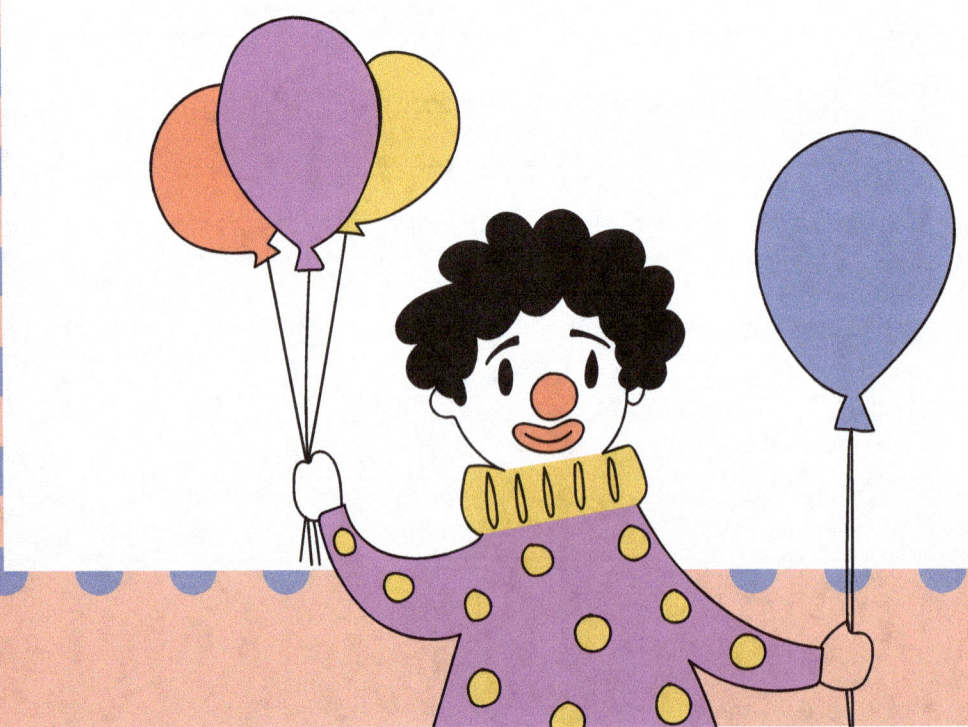

Answer the questions in complete sentences.

1. What day did Jonathan go to the circus and with whom?

_____

_____

_____

2. What was the first thing Jonathan saw when he entered the circus?

_____

_____

_____

3. What did Jonathan see at the circus and what did he like best?

_____

_____

_____

_____

_____

4. Why do you think the audience was breathless as they watched the acrobat?

_____

_____

_____

_____

_____

_____

Read the texts and answer the questions in complete sentences.

Moving out

John is an eight-year-old boy who has lived his whole life in the city. The houses were attached, there were many cars, and the noise was never-ending. But John liked the city a lot because that's where all his friends lived, where his school and favorite park that he went to every afternoon was. The day his mom announced that they were moving to the village, he was sure he wouldn't like it at all and was very sad.

When they arrived at their new house the first thing that struck John was the large garden. There was a huge garden at the back of the house full of flowers and trees! The house was quite a bit bigger than the one he had in the city. It had two large bedrooms, a spacious kitchen, a small sitting room, and a large living room. "I'm going to have a great birthday party here!" he thought as soon as he saw his new home.

A few days later, John met new friends in the neighborhood and started spending more time outside playing and exploring. A month later, John realized the change was better than expected.

Answer the questions in complete sentences.

1. How old was John and where did he live his whole life?

_____

_____

2. How did he react when he found out about the move?
Why do you think he felt that way?

_____

_____

_____

_____

3. Describe John's new house and garden.

_____

_____

_____

_____

4. What changed for John after the move?

_____

_____

_____

_____

_____

5. How does he feel about the change now?

_____

_____

_____

_____

_____

6. Where would you like to live? In the city or the village, and why?

_____

_____

_____

_____

_____

_____

_____

128

Read the texts and answer the questions in complete sentences.

Vacation on a magical island

As the summer began, my anticipation for the holidays was building. This year, my family had decided we were going to Santorini. I had seen so many pictures and heard countless stories about how breathtaking this island can be, and I was really looking forward to our vacation.

As we arrived, I was instantly enchanted by the view of the sea, all the shades of blue before us, creating the perfect contrast with the island's white houses. Walking along the narrow alleys, we discovered little corners with local delicacies and shops with handmade jewelry. In the afternoons, we cherished the magical sunsets as the red and orange color of the setting sun reflected on the deep blue sea.

Over the next few days, our island tours continued to amaze us. We visited Akrotiri, where we admired the archaeological finds and learned about the area's ancient history. We also and went on a boat ride around the islets, where we dived in the turquoise waters. On one of our tours, we were stunned by the red beach with its colored rocks and the wonderful sound of the waves.

As always, the vacation seemed to end very quickly. It was hard to say goodbye to this beautiful island, but we were sure that the memories we collected would keep us company for a long time.

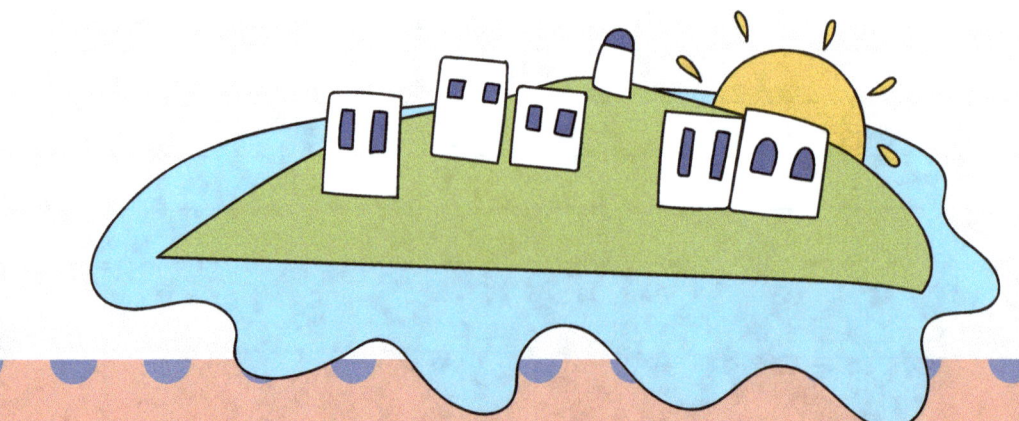

© Upbility

Answer the questions in complete sentences.

1. Where did the child's family go on vacation this summer?

_____

_____

2. What color were the houses on the island?

_____

_____

3. How did they spend their afternoons on the island?

_____

_____

_____

_____

_____

_____

_____

4. How did you spend your summer vacation?

_____

_____

_____

_____

_____

_____

_____

_____

_____

_____

Read the texts and answer the questions in complete sentences.

A funny incident

It was a summer Saturday morning, and the Johnson family had woken up early, getting ready for a long trip to the mountains. Before they set off, Elijah, the family's eldest son, and his little sister, Amelia, decided to make breakfast for everyone.

They had in mind to make pancakes with honey and fruit. While Elijah rummaged through the cupboards for the ingredients, Amelia prepared the pan and the plates. But in haste, Elijah grabbed the salt instead of sugar! They put all the ingredients in a bowl and mixed them together until they made a nice dough.

When it was time to pour the mixture into the pan, the wonderful aroma of pancakes filled the house. Everyone sat down at the table, excited. Dad was the first to taste the pancakes, and his eyes rolled! Mom and Elijah had the same reaction when they tasted them next.

"What's wrong with pancakes? They're so salty!" said the mother. Amelia looked at the jar they used and realized the mistake. Everyone burst out laughing!

In the end, the family enjoyed some yogurt with fresh fruit. This family breakfast would surely be something to laugh about for years to come!

Answer the questions in complete sentences.

1. What had the Johnson family planned to do on Saturday morning?

_____

_____

_____

_____

2. What did the children do wrong while preparing the pancakes?

_____

_____

_____

_____

3. Who tasted the pancakes first and how did they react?

_____

_____

_____

_____

4. What did the family decide to eat after they realized the mistake?

_____

_____

_____

_____

5. Describe a funny incident you had with your family!

_____

_____

_____

_____

_____

_____

_____

_____

Read the texts and answer the questions in complete sentences.

A visit to the public library

Eleanor and George, two friends from school, had heard of their town's public library many times but had never visited it. Today, they decided to go finally.

Outside the library they were struck by the imposing building; up close it was even more impressive. Once through the large wooden door, they first noticed the high ceiling with its carved columns and the colorful glass that strangely reflected the sunlight on the floor. The atmosphere was calm and relaxing, with sounds of whispers and turning pages.

In one corner, there was the children's section. Kids of various ages sat on small couches and did puzzles or read stories and literature while a nice librarian recommended books to other kids and their parents.

George, who loved science, found a book about the universe, while Eleanor, who liked fairy tales, chose a book full of stories about mythical heroes, spells, and adventures. The library also had a digital corner where children could listen to recorded fairy tales or play educational computer games. The two friends were delighted by these activities and they decided to spend most of their time there.

The afternoon passed quickly, and when it was time to leave, Eleanor and George were holding the books they had chosen. With smiles on their faces, they promised to return soon to this wondrous place of knowledge and imagination.

Answer the questions in complete sentences.

1. Who are the two protagonists of the story and how do they know each other?

_____

_____

2. What struck them and what did the children first notice
when they entered the library?

_____

_____

_____

_____

3. Which part of the library did the children like best?

_____

_____

_____

_____

4. Which book did the boy choose and which book did the girl choose?

_____

_____

_____

_____

5. Do you think the children liked the library? How could you tell?

_____

_____

_____

_____

_____

_____

_____

_____

Read the texts and answer the questions in complete sentences.

The parade

It was a sunny morning and Nick woke up early, eager for the big day. He was very proud to be watching the parade this year. He had put on his white shirt, black trousers, and shiniest belt.

As he walked with his classmates down the main street, he noticed many families already seated in the front row waiting for the parade to begin. Nick's grandmother, Mrs. Helen, was there and smiled warmly at him.

The street was filled with the melodies of the philharmonic orchestra. Nick was impressed by the military vehicles, but his favorite part was when a group of child scouts flew white and blue balloons into the sky, creating a beautiful sight.

In the end, the day was full of joy, music, and color. As Nick returned home, full of beautiful images, he wondered what it would be like to participate actively in next year's parade.

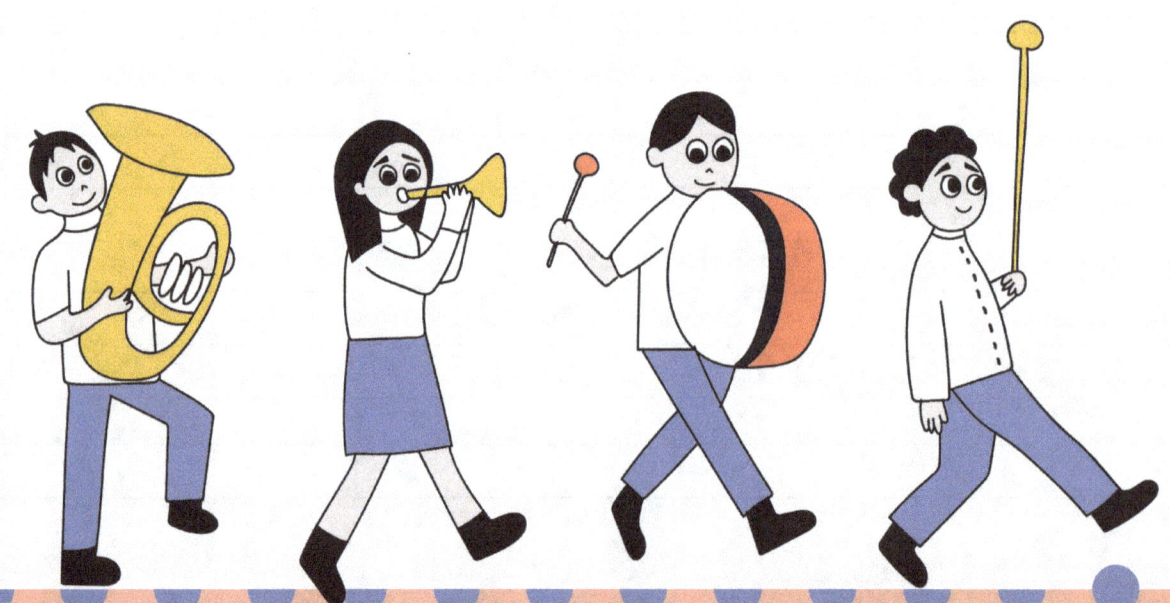

Answer the questions in complete sentences.

1. Why did Nick wake up impatient? What was special about this day?

_____

_____

_____

_____

2. Which relative had Nick seen at the parade?

_____

_____

3. How did Nick dress?

_____

_____

_____

_____

4. Which part of the parade did Nick like best?

_____

_____

_____

_____

5. What did Nick think at the end of the day?

_____

_____

_____

_____

_____

_____

Read the texts and answer the questions in complete sentences.

The new student

It was the third week of September when Jim noticed an unfamiliar student sitting at the last desk in the second row. George, a boy with bright brown eyes and brown hair, was the new kid in the class. As soon as Mrs. Olivia entered the classroom she introduced him to everyone, and they all said their names one by one. He had recently moved to town because of his father's job, who was in the military.

Jim noticed how nervously George played with his pencil during the first hour. During the recess, he approached George and welcomed him. Together, they walked through the schoolyard, eating their sandwiches, and Jim showed George the herb garden that their class had planted and was in charge of. He then reintroduced him to all his classmates.

George told Jim about his old town and his school, how much he missed his friends and the games they played. However, he liked the idea of meeting new friends and learning new games.

During the following recesses, George showed his talent for soccer. Jim and the rest of his classmates really admired him and all the kids wanted him on their team. After that, George quickly became very popular among his classmates!

In the evening, George was very happy about his new school and his new friends. He had a lot to tell his family. While George's day started with a lot of stress, it ended with laughter, games, and new friendships.

Answer the questions in complete sentences. :

1. Why did George move to the city?

_____

_____

2. How did George feel at the beginning of the day?
Why do you think he had these feelings?

_____

_____

_____

_____

_____

3. How did George spend his first recess at his new school?

_____

_____

_____

4. What was George talented at?

_____

_____

5. How did George feel at the end of the school day?

_____

_____

_____

_____

_____

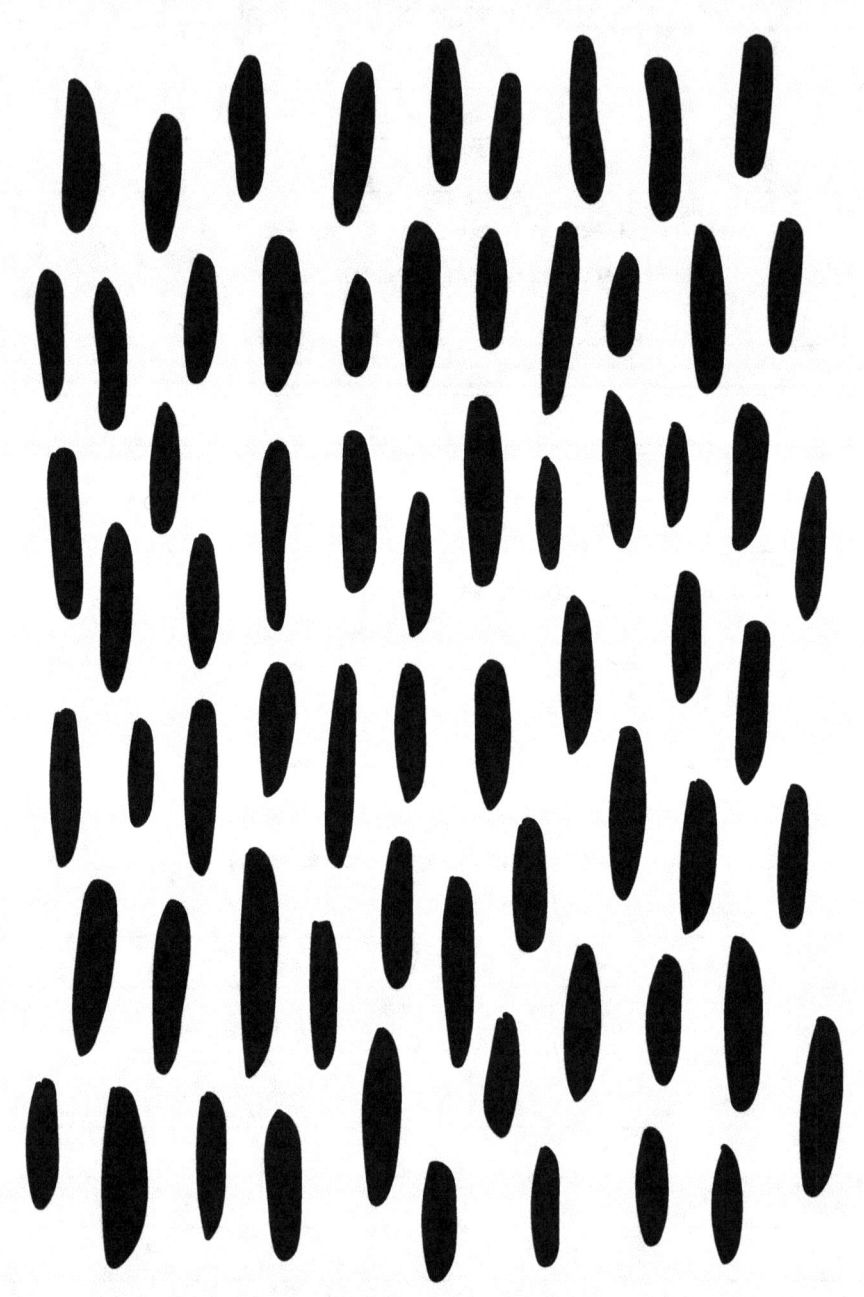

LEVEL 6

Read the texts carefully and solve the exercises.

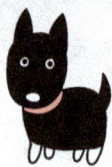

Playing with Zuzu

Sebastian and Evelyn play with their dog, Zuzu, in the yard. It's a bright and sunny day. They spend hours playing ball and chasing each other. Zuzu loves spending time with the kids, she seems very happy and jumps all the time.

After playing, they eat ice cream in the shade of a tree. It's their favorite part of their day!

Mark the following sentences as True or False.

The day is sunny and bright. _____

The children and the dog spend hours playing hide and seek. _____

Zuzu is angry that the children won't give her ice cream. _____

Choose the correct answer.

Zuzu is a:

A) Cat
B) Dog
C) Parrot

What they eat after playing:

A) Candy
B) Chocolate
C) Ice cream

Answer the question in a complete sentence.

1. What is the children's favorite part of the day?

_____

_____

_____

_____

_____

_____

2. Make a drawing that's related to the text.

Read the texts carefully and solve the exercises.

A day without school

Such a day would be very special because there would be no alarm clocks and no morning rush. You could stay in bed a little longer, stretch your arms and legs, and relax in bed as much as you want. When you get up, you'll have the whole day ahead of you to do the things you love and more importantly, you won't have homework for the afternoon!

On a day like this, the possibilities are endless. You can play with your favorite toys, make crafts, read a favorite book, or even help out with cooking. You can also go out to play in the park or go for a bike ride. This day is the perfect opportunity to do whatever makes you happy and get some rest so you're ready for the following days at school and full of energy!

Mark the following sentences as True or False.

On a day without school, you rush out of

bed to enjoy your day.   _____

When you don't go to school, you have time to

do the activities you like.   _____

A day without school is a good opportunity to rest.   _____

Choose the correct answer.

According to the text, what can you do in a day without school?

A) Go shopping

B) Play with your toys

C) Clean the garden

Where can you go to play outside on a day without school?

A) To the park

B) To the shopping center

C) To Godmother's house

Answer in a complete sentence.

Describe how you would like to spend a day without school.

_____

_____

_____

_____

_____

_____

_____

_____

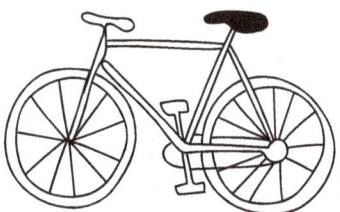

Read the texts carefully and solve the exercises.

The neighbor's dog

Next to our house lives Mr. Samuel and his family. Mr. Samuel has a playful little dog, Luki. Luki is a small dog with white and brown fur, brown shiny eyes, and a black nose that sneaks around and sniffs everything!

Every morning when I go to school, I see him playing in the garden, running after the butterflies and perking up his ears whenever he hears a strange noise. Luki always looks happy and ready to play. Mr. Samuel told me that if he gives someone his ball, it means he wants to be his friend, and he has given it to me!

Luki seems to love kids a lot. As soon as a child approaches him, he starts wagging his tail and twirling around like he's dancing. When Luki does tricks, all the kids in the neighborhood clap and laugh. He has become everyone's favorite friend in the neighborhood and we are all very happy to have him around.

Mark the following sentences as True or False.

Luki is a big dog. _____

The neighbor's dog plays in the garden every morning. _____

Luki doesn't like being around children. _____

Choose the correct answer.

What color is Luki's fur?

A) Black and white
B) White and brown
C) Brown and black
D) White and grey

What does Luki do when he hears a strange noise?

A) He plays with his ball

B) He lifts up his ears

C) He runs

D) He twirls around like he's dancing

Why are the children clapping for Luki?

A) Because he gives them his ball

B) Because he brings them their slippers

C) Because he does tricks

D) Because he runs after the butterflies

Answer the following questions in complete sentences.

1. What does Luki look like?

_____

_____

_____

_____

_____

2. What does Luki do when he wants to be friends with a child?

_____

_____

_____

_____

_____

Read the texts carefully and solve the exercises.

My favorite toy

My favorite toy is a small, electronic car, which is bright red and black with sparkly wheels. I got this little car last year for my birthday as a gift from my parents, and it has been a favorite toy ever since. It has a small motor inside that makes it run really fast, and I can control it with a remote control. I love it so much because my parents got it for me and because I'm the first among my friends to have a little car like this. It makes me feel very special.

I usually play with my little car every weekend along with my brother and neighborhood friends on our spare time. Everyone loves watching the little car do amazing tricks and overcome obstacles. Sometimes, we have races and contests to see which little car is the fastest or who can do the best tricks. My toy car is the most fun toy I've ever had and I hope to have it for many years to come.

Mark the following sentences as True or False.

The child's favorite toy is a big electronic car. _____

The car is red and black. _____

The car is controlled by remote control. _____

Choose the correct answer.

When does the child usually play with his favorite toy?

A) Every day after school
B) Every weekend
C) Only on weekdays

With whom does the child play with his favorite toy?

A) With his parents

B) With his brother

C) With his brother and his friends

What do the child and his friends do with the toy cars?

A) They line them up

B) They organize races

C) They wash them

Answer the following questions in complete sentences.

1. Why is the car his favorite toy?

_____

_____

_____

_____

_____

2. What is your favorite toy and why?

_____

_____

_____

_____

_____

_____

Read the texts carefully and solve the exercises.

A family trip

Last Sunday, my family and I went on a wonderful trip to the mountains. I was very excited because I love nature trips, so I woke up very early in the morning. Mom had already prepared the sandwiches, and Dad loaded the car with water, juice, and fruits. I made sure to bring a ball, a board game, and our little dog, Zuzu.

When we reached the mountain, we were stunned by the magnificent view. The birds were tweeting sweetly, and the trees were so tall they almost touched the clouds. We walked through paths of blooming flowers and played hide and seek and ball with Zuzu. Zuzu's joy couldn't be hidden. She kept running up and down and wagging her tail, as this was the first time she had so much room to run. Afterward, we sat in a beautiful green meadow for a picnic and enjoyed our sandwiches and fruit.

This day was truly wonderful. We saw colorful butterflies and wildflowers. We even saw a rare flower species, and Dad explained that it's endangered and that we were very lucky to have seen it! In the afternoon, we played a game called "Guess the Animal" and had a great laugh at Dad's funny imitations. On the way home I was very tired and slept in the car. This family trip was one of the best trips I have taken with my family.

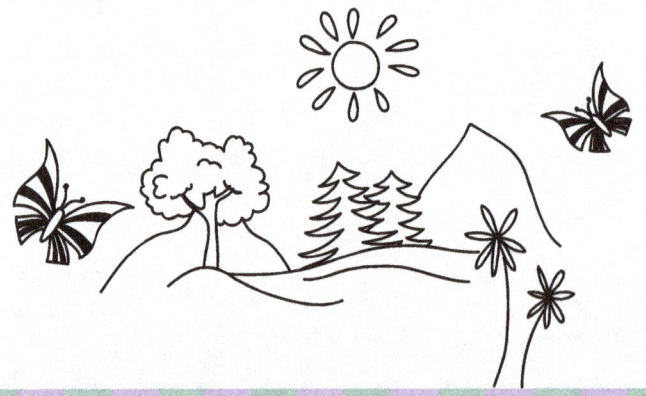

Mark the following sentences as True or False.

The family went on a trip to the sea.   _____

The family's little dog went with them on the trip.   _____

The family played hide and seek and ball.   _____

The trip was frustrating and tiring for the child.   _____

Choose the correct answer.

Where did the family go on a trip?

A) To the mountain
B) To the beach
C) To a theme park

What did the child take with him on the trip?

A) A book and a ball
B) His favorite ball and a board game
C) A toy and a book

What did the family eat at the picnic?

A) Pizza
B) Sandwiches and fruit
C) Hamburger

What game did they play at the end of the trip?

A) Monopoly
B) Guess the animal
C) Chess

Answer the following questions in complete sentences.

1. If you could add one more thing to the day, what would it be and why?

_____

_____

_____

_____

_____

2. Describe a trip you took with your family.

_____

_____

_____

_____

_____

_____

_____

_____

_____

_____

_____

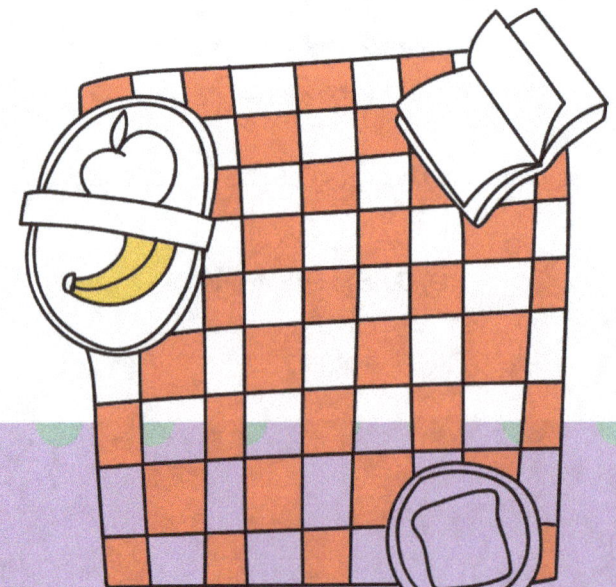

Read the texts carefully and solve the exercises.

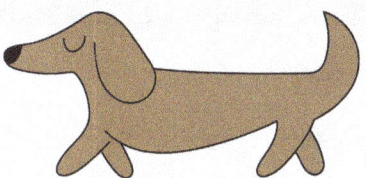

Leo's accident

On Sunday morning, Leo decided to try out his new bike that his uncle had given him for his birthday. It was blue, with bright yellow stripes, and had a little bell on the handlebars. He put on his new superhero hat that his grandmother had given him and started his long ride.

Leo was happily pedaling through the park when one of his favorite songs was playing on an ice cream vendor's vehicle. He stopped for an ice cream and to listen to his favorite song better. Unfortunately, at the same time, a small dog with brown fur and a puffy tail was crossing the street to go to the other side of the park.

In his attempt to avoid the little dog, Leo lost his balance and fell into the grass. His bicycle rolled a few feet away. He stood up cautiously when he realized that his new hat was stained by ice cream thrown on the ground.

Although he was a little scared, he was fine. The little dog approached him, licking his hand as if to apologize. Leo petted it and laughed while a girl who saw what happened gave him a tissue. Within minutes, the fear was gone and Leo was back on his feet with a new four-legged friend by his side.

Mark the following sentences as True or False.

Leo got the bike as an Easter present.　　　　　　　　_____

Leo's bike is blue with yellow stripes.　　　　　　　_____

Leo stopped to buy water from the ice cream seller.　_____

A little dog ran in front of Leo as he pedaled.　　　_____

Choose the correct answer.

What color was Leo's bike?

A) Red
B) Blue
C) Green

Why did Leo approach the ice cream seller?

A) He wanted to get water
B) He wanted to get juice
C) He wanted to listen to the song

Answer the following questions in complete sentences.

1. What was Leo's reaction when the dog approached him
after the accident?

_____

_____

_____

_____

_____

2. How do you think Leo felt about his bike and his hat?

_____

_____

_____

_____

_____

_____

_____

_____

Put the events below in the correct order according to the text.

⇨ The little dog approached him and licked his hand.

_____

⇨ Leo had decided to try out his new bike.

_____

⇨ Leo's favorite song started playing on an ice cream
   vendor's vehicle.

_____

⇨ Leo was happily pedaling through the park.

_____

⇨ Leo fell on the grass.

_____

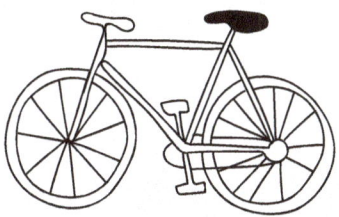

A unique ride with the bike

On Saturday morning, Sebastian decided to go for a ride with his bike. It was a bike with little bells and colored stickers that glowed in the sun. He was very happy because he had several commitments all week and didn't have time to ride his bike in the afternoons. He had recently moved with his family to the neighborhood and hadn't had much time to explore it.

The road led him to a beautiful park full of blossoming trees and colorful lilacs. The birds were chirping and reminded him that spring was already here. Soon, he found a path that led to a small forest of dense pine trees.

As he passed through the forest, he noticed a soft rainbow forming in one part of the sky, "It's raining somewhere nearby," he thought and smiled. Sebastian stopped for a moment, got off his bike, and looked at the rainbow in admiration. It was probably the last one he would see this year since summer would be here in a few days.

He continued his ride and passed by a house where some children played in the garden. The children saw Sebastian and invited him to a bike race, which he gladly accepted. Laughter and shouts echoed in the air as the young cyclists raced and then went for their ride.

Time was ticking away and Sebastian had to get home, it was already midday. This morning was what he really needed after a hard week.

Mark the following sentences as True or False.

Sebastian took his ride in the summer. _____

Sebastian's bike had colored bells. _____

Sebastian had a bike race with his friends. _____

Sebastian recently moved into the neighborhood. _____

On his ride, Sebastian saw a rainbow. _____

Sebastian went for a ride on his bike every afternoon that week. _____

Choose the correct answer.

Where did the road lead Sebastian on his bike ride?

A) To a shopping mall

B) To a park with blossoming trees

C) To a theme park

D) To his school

What did Sebastian do when he saw the rainbow?

A) He kept riding his bike faster

B) He went to find its end

C) He stopped to admire it

D) He took a picture

When did Sebastian return home?

A) Morning

B) Noon

C) Afternoon

D) Evening

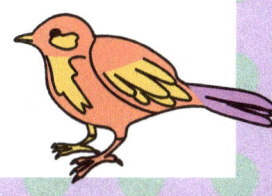

Answer the following questions in complete sentences.

1. Why was Sebastian so eager to go for a walk on Saturday morning?

_____

_____

_____

_____

_____

2. How do you usually spend your Saturday mornings?

_____

_____

_____

_____

_____

_____

_____

_____

Put the events below in the correct order according to the text.

⇨ He went to a park with blossoming trees where birds were singing.   _____

⇨ He found himself in a small forest.   _____

⇨ He had a bike race with some children he met.   _____

⇨ He admired the rainbow.   _____

⇨ He left his house on his bike.   _____

⇨ He followed a path.   _____

Read the texts carefully and solve the exercises.

Carnival Parade

The day that both kids and grownups had been waiting for had arrived! It was the day of the big carnival parade and the whole town had been on its feet since morning. The main square was filled with stalls selling confetti and masks. The carnival music played early on the town's speakers while children and their parents gathered to watch the parade, dance, and have fun.

Everyone watching the parade was dressed up. Some disguised themselves as unrecognizable, while others chose something small and subtle, like a mask or hat. One thing's for sure! You couldn't tell who was young and old inside all those costumes.

The parade started with the town cantors, who rode on a moving platform pulled by a car. The cheerleaders and dancers followed. Then, many small and large floats appeared, each with a different theme: the world of the sea, famous explorers, superheroes, and many others that made the children cheer in admiration. Several themes poked fun at everyday life and politics, providing laughs, especially for the adults. Among the floats, clowns, stilt walkers, and jugglers passed by doing funny tricks and making animals out of balloons.

At the end of the parade, the city's mayor handed out prizes for the most original costumes and the most impressive floats. Young and old who participated felt proud of their effort and creativity.

The parade ended, but the laughter and memories remained, with the promise that next year's carnival parade would be even more exciting.

Mark the following sentences as True or False.

The whole city eagerly awaited the carnival parade.   _____

The parade began with the cantors singing as they walked.   _____

There were floats with a superhero theme.   _____

Those watching the parade were dressed up.   _____

The Mayor handed out awards at the end of the parade.   _____

Choose the correct answer.

Where did the Carnival parade take place?

A) At the school

B) In the main square

C) In an event hall

D) In a park

What is not mentioned as part of the parade?

A) Floats

B) Jugglers

C) School band

D) Clowns

Which of the following was the subject of one of the floats?

A) The world of the sea

B) Famous musicians

C) Astronauts

D) Fantastic creatures

What did the parents do during the parade?

A) Leading the floats

B) Escorting their children in costume

C) Playing music

D) Selling tickets

Answer the following questions in complete sentences.

1. How did the children who participated in the parade feel?

_____
_____
_____
_____
_____
_____

2. What did the jugglers do during the parade?

_____
_____
_____
_____
_____
_____

Put the events below in the correct order according to the text.

⇨ The Mayor awarded the prizes. _____

⇨ The children put on their costumes. _____

⇨ The dancers paraded. _____

⇨ Young and old gathered in the main square. _____

⇨ The cantors started the parade. _____

⇨ Jugglers made balloons for the children. _____

Read the texts carefully and solve the exercises.

A fight at school

A few days ago, something happened in my classroom that really bothered me. It was a fight between two of my classmates, George and Nick. It all started with a game at recess. George and Nick started arguing about who won the football game and slowly their disagreement turned into a fight. They started shouting at each other and using bad words. The game was forgotten and now everyone was watching the two friends fighting.

The teachers immediately separated them, trying to figure out what happened. After a while, they both calmed down and started talking about the incident. They realized that their fight started over a minor thing and that they lost control. Our teacher explained to them how important it is to communicate better and not let our anger get the better of us. She talked to us about the importance of patience and understanding the feelings of others. After George and Nick calmed down, they realized their fight was pointless. They apologized to each other and decided to forget about their disagreement.

This fight showed all the children how easy it is for two friends to misunderstand each other and how misunderstandings can be solved with patience and understanding. In the following days when several disagreements arose, we all managed them with patience and communication, so there were no more fights in the group.

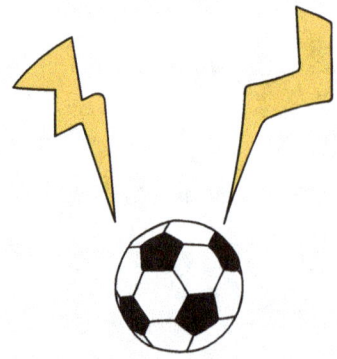

Mark the following sentences as True or False.

George and Nick used bad words about each other. _____

The teachers were not involved at all during the fight. _____

George and Nick disagreed about one important reason. _____

After the fight, George and Nick apologized to each other. _____

Choose the correct answer.

What caused the initial disagreement between George and Nick?

A. A school lesson

B. A football game

C. An answer to an exercise

How did the teachers react to the fight?

A. They let them solve the argument on their own

B. They separated them and talked to them

C. They gave them more homework

What did the student telling the story learn from this fight?

A. How to avoid fights

B. How to be right after a fight

C. How to resolve disagreements

Answer the following questions in complete sentences.

1. Do you think the teacher's intervention was important? Why?

_____

_____

_____

_____

_____

_____

_____

2. How would you deal with a misunderstanding or a fight with a classmate? What do you think are the best tactics to resolve a disagreement?

_____

_____

_____

_____

_____

_____

_____

_____

_____

_____

_____

_____

_____

Read the texts carefully and solve the exercises.

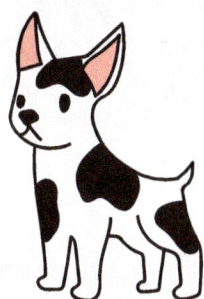

The dog shelter

In a small village just outside the city, there was a dog shelter. The shelter was like a big house with many yards where the dogs could run and play. Kevin, a fourteen-year-old volunteer, loved to spend his free time there taking care of the dogs.

Every day after school, Kevin would go to the shelter. The first thing he did was feed the dogs. Then, he would take them out one by one for a walk in the village. The dogs loved the walks and Kevin because they felt his love and care.

One afternoon, Kevin noticed a new dog in the shelter, a small dog with white and black fur. The dog looked scared and shy. Kevin decided to spend more time with him, trying to make him feel safe.

Day by day, the dog began to overcome his fear. He started playing with the other dogs and waiting for Kevin at the door every afternoon. Kevin was very happy that this little dog had adapted to the shelter.

The dog shelter was not just a place for stray dogs to find a home. It was also a place where people could learn about the importance of care, love, and loyalty, like Kevin.

Mark the following sentences as True or False.

The dog shelter is located in the city center. _____

Kevin is a volunteer and spends his free time taking
care of the dogs at the shelter. _____

Kevin feeds the dogs and only takes them for walks
on the weekends. _____

At the shelter, there are many yards and areas where
the dogs can play. _____

Kevin was initially scared of the dogs. _____

Choose the correct answer.

Where is the dog shelter located?

A) In the city center

B) Near the sea

C) Near the forest

D) In a small village

How old is Kevin?

A) 10 years old

B) 12 years old

C) 14 years old

D) 16 years old

What does Kevin do when he arrives at the shelter?

A) He plays with the dogs

B) He feeds the dogs

C) He reads books

D) He helps with the cleaning

What was the new dog's reaction when he saw Kevin?

A) He was excited

B) He was scared

C) He was indifferent

D) He barked aggressively

What did Kevin learn at the shelter?

A) Survival techniques

B) The importance of care and love

C) How to drive

D) History of dogs

Answer the following questions in complete sentences.

1. Why did Kevin decide to spend more time with the new dog?

_____

_____

_____

_____

_____

2. How did the new dog's behavior change after he started spending time with Kevin?

_____

_____

_____

_____

_____

Put the events below in the correct order according to the text.

⇨ Kevin notices a new dog in the shelter.   _____

⇨ Kevin decides to spend more time with the new dog.   _____

⇨ The new dog begins to play with the other dogs.   _____

⇨ Kevin arrives at the shelter and begins to feed the dogs. _____

⇨ Kevin is happy about the dog's adjustment.

Read the texts carefully and solve the exercises.

What I want to be when I grow up

When I was little, they asked me what I wanted to be when I grew up, and I always gave two answers: a footballer or a doctor. The last two years I don't want either, because I learned about astronauts. I want to be an astronaut now so I can travel deep into space, explore unknown planets, and see the stars up close. I believe it's one of the most exciting and adventurous professions in the world.

Unfortunately, becoming an astronaut is not easy. It takes a lot of hard work and a lot of studying! You have to be very good at sciences like physics and mathematics. You also have to be very fit and keep your body healthy, and of course, you have to be ready to face challenges. Astronauts spend many hours in training to learn how to survive for months in space and work there.

One of the reasons I like the idea of being an astronaut is that you are part of space exploration and contribute to scientific knowledge and new discoveries.

I imagine myself looking at the Earth from afar and feeling a sense of wonder at the beauty of the universe.

Becoming an astronaut is a dream worth pursuing. It's a profession that combines adventure, science, and exploration. It offers a unique experience that you can't find in any other profession!

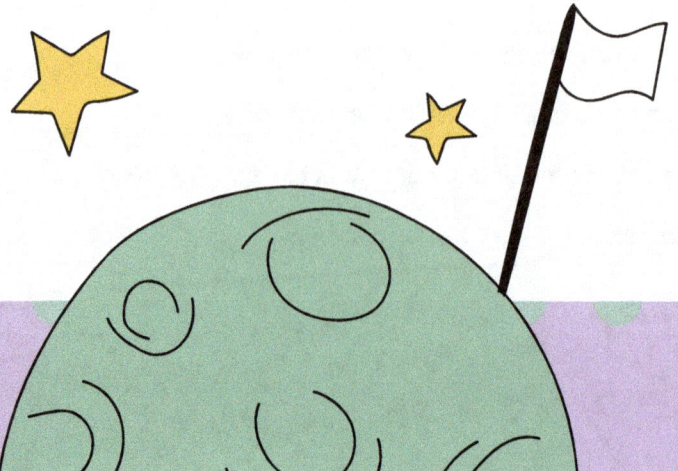

Mark the following sentences as True or False.

The author wanted to be an astronaut from a young age.   _____

To be an astronaut, you don't have to be fit.   _____

Astronauts spend many hours in training.   _____

Being an astronaut is interesting because you contribute
to scientific knowledge.   _____

Choose the correct answer.

Which science is essential for someone who wants to become an astronaut?

A) History

B) Physics

C) Philosophy

D) Literature

What feeling does the author describe when imagining seeing Earth from space?

A) Fear

B) Indifference

C) Admiration

D) Sadness

What is the main reason the author wants to become an astronaut?

A) To become famous

B) For adventure and exploration

C) To earn a lot of money

D) Because they like space movies

Which of the following is not a requirement to become an astronaut?

A) Good physical fitness
B) Education in science
C) Knowledge of cooking
D) Training for space

Answer the following questions in complete sentences.

1. Why does the child want to be an astronaut?

_____

_____

_____

_____

_____

_____

2. Based on the text and your own knowledge,
write down a negative aspect of being an astronaut.

_____

_____

_____

_____

_____

_____

_____

_____

_____

3. What do you want to be when you grow up?

_____
_____
_____
_____
_____
_____
_____
_____
_____
_____
_____
_____
_____
_____
_____

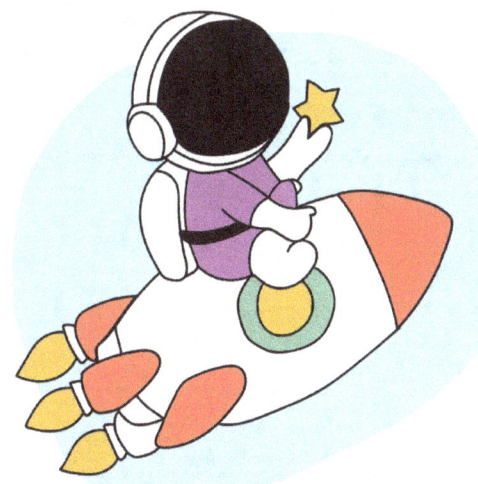

Read the texts carefully and solve the exercises.

The lost key

One day, when I came home from school, I realized I had lost my house's key. It was a small key that my mom had put in a little bag inside my backpack so I could get into the house by myself. At first, I wasn't too worried. I thought maybe I had put it somewhere else.

I started looking everywhere. I looked in all the pockets of my bag, in the pockets of my trousers, even under the garden furniture, to see if it had fallen as I opened the bag. But the key was nowhere. I felt a lot of anxiety because the key wasn't just an object, it represented the trust that my family had shown me.

Finally, I decided to follow the route to school, just in case I had dropped it somewhere. I remembered that I had walked my friend George to his house and then stopped by the park to see the new equipment they had installed and had sat on a bench for a while. I went everywhere, but unfortunately I couldn't find it.

I had now given up hope of finding the little bag with the key when I thought I would stop by the school to check around the classroom. Once I got to the school entrance, I saw Mrs. Georgia, who cleans our school, sweeping the yard. I ran over to her and asked her permission to go to my classroom and look for my key. Then, she pulled my little bag out of her pocket with a calm smile! She had found it when she was sweeping my classroom. I immediately felt an incredible relief. It was like finding a treasure.

This experience made me realize that I need to be more careful and responsible for things people entrust to me.

Mark the following sentences as True or False.

The student found the key in his bag. _____

The student lost the key on his way to school. _____

The lost key was found under a bush in the park. _____

The student felt relieved when he found the key. _____

The child at school met his teacher. _____

Choose the correct answer.

Where did the student start looking for the lost key?

A) In the park

B) At school

C) In his yard

D) At his friend's house

What did the student feel when he realized that the key was lost?

A) Excitement

B) Fear

C) Relief

D) Anxiety

What does the key symbolize to the student?

A) A simple object

B) The trust of his family

C) A toy

D) An opportunity for adventure

Finally, the key was found:

A) In his backyard

B) In the school

C) In the park

D) At his friend's house

Answer the following questions in complete sentences.

1. How do you think the student would feel if he didn't find the key?

_____
_____
_____
_____

2. Describe an incident in which you lost something important to you. What was it? How did you feel and why?

_____
_____
_____
_____
_____
_____
_____
_____
_____

Put the events below in the correct order according to the text.

⇨ The student discovered that the key was lost.   _____

⇨ He went to look for it in the park.   _____

⇨ The student returned home from school.   _____

⇨ He felt relieved when he found the key.   _____

⇨ He went to look on the way to his friend's house.   _____

⇨ He began to look for the key everywhere in the backyard.   _____

⇨ He went to look for it at school.   _____

⇨ Mrs. Georgia gave him the bag with the key in it.   _____

Read the texts carefully and solve the exercises.

A different birthday gift

Sunday would have been Maria's birthday. Her friends and family were thinking about what gift to give her. Maria hadn't asked for anything in particular, but everyone knew she loved stories and adventures. So they decided to give her a different gift than usual: a beautiful adventure that would give her lots of stories to enjoy!

On Sunday afternoon, Maria eagerly awaited what they had planned for her. Once everyone was gathered at her house, she opened the only present in front of her with great anticipation. Inside, she found a small box. In the box, there was a map and a letter that said: "Your adventure begins." Maria was thrilled with the idea of a hidden treasure!

She and her friends started to follow the map. Each point on the map led them to different places in the city, where they had to solve various puzzles to move on to the next point. They went to the park, the school, the main square, Uncle Greg's house, and the local bakery. The final stop was the garden of her house. Digging behind the lemon tree, she discovered a box filled with literary books and a note from her friends and relatives saying: "Every day you read, you live a new adventure." It was the most unusual yet perfect gift she could have received.

Now, every night before she goes to sleep, Maria travels to distant lands and has countless adventures. It was one of the most beautiful birthdays for her. The hidden treasure hunt gave her many stories to discover in those books!

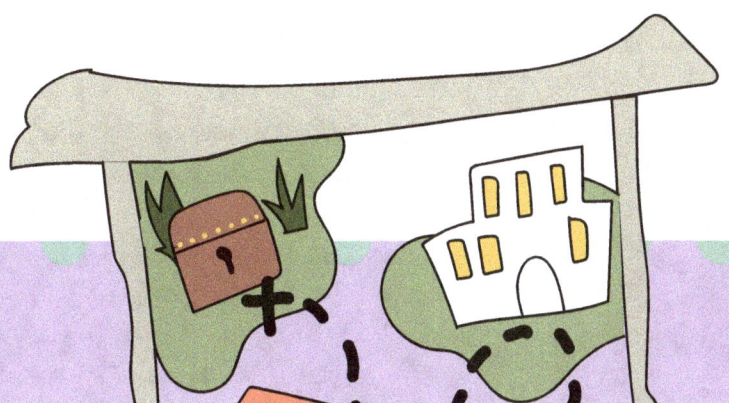

Mark the following sentences as True or False.

Maria asked for a specific gift for her birthday.   _____

Maria's birthday was on Saturday.   _____

The final stop for the lost treasure was the neighborhood bakery.   _____

The box was buried behind a lemon tree.   _____

Maria's gift was the map of a hidden treasure.   _____

Choose the correct answer.

When did everyone gather for Maria's birthday?

A) Morning

B) Noon

C) Afternoon

D) Evening

What was finally Maria's gift?

A) A toy

B) A bicycle

C) A box of books

D) A box of toys

How did Maria feel when she received her gift?

A) Disappointed

B) Excited

C) Indifferent

D) Sad

What was the message on the note left by Maria's parents?

A) "We bought you the most beautiful books."

B) "Your adventure begins."

C) "Every day you read, you live a new adventure."

D) "We hope you like your presents."

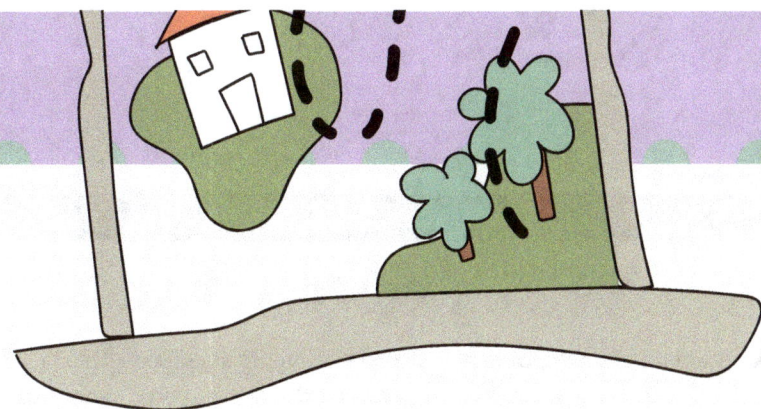

Answer the following questions in complete sentences.

1. What did Maria do every night before she went to sleep after her birthday?

_____

_____

_____

_____

_____

2. What made Maria's gift different and special?

_____

_____

_____

_____

_____

Put the events below in the correct order according to the text.

⇨ Maria found many books in a box.   _____

⇨ Maria was looking forward to her birthday present.   _____

⇨ The Hidden Treasure began!   _____

⇨ She dug in the garden of her house.   _____

⇨ Maria had many adventures through the books before she went to sleep. _____

⇨ She solved many puzzles in different places in the city.   _____

Read the texts carefully and solve the exercises.

The big secret

There was a distant, beautiful, and cold village called Love. The inhabitants there had a strange tradition: every year, each child turning nine years old undertook a great mission to discover "The Big Secret." No one knew what it was since those who discovered it never talked about it, and everyone claimed it was something that changed their lives forever.

This year, little Helen turns nine and it's her turn to discover the Big Secret. On the day of her birthday, the village Leader handed her an old map and a wooden rosary with nine beads. "Follow the map and count the beads. In the end, you will find the big secret," he told her, smiling broadly.

Helen, holding the rosary tightly in her hand, began her adventure. She passed through valleys and streams, crossed a lush green forest, and followed the song of birds that led her to a hidden blue lake. There, she had to solve a riddle that would open the way to the big secret.

The riddle required her to think of all the qualities every person needs to live by. Helen initially found it very difficult because she didn't know how many of these qualities there might be. Then she remembered the words of the village Leader. She counted the beads of the rosary. There were nine beads, so she decided to find nine values. Each bead represented a virtue; she thought of generosity, truth, courage, friendship, and other precious values that Helen had learned and was trying to cultivate in her life. With the help of these virtues, she solved the puzzle and the lake formed a stream that led her to a beautiful green valley.

In the heart of the valley was a towering cypress tree, and beneath it, a manuscript said: "The great secret is nothing but the discovery of your virtues and the wisdom to live by them every day." Helen understood then that the great secret is realizing the values she has in her life and deciding to always uphold them.

She returned to the village happy, ready to share with others not the details of the secret but the wisdom and knowledge she had gained. The great secret continued to live on in the hearts of all as a promise of a life full of great virtues and valuable lessons.

Mark the following sentences as True or False.

Helen had to discover the big secret before she was nine years old. _____

The Leader gave Helen an old map and a rosary for her mission. _____

Helen went through a secret forest to find the hidden lake. _____

The lake was the final point of the quest for the Big Secret. _____

The Big Secret was a treasure full of beads and gems. _____

Choose the correct answer.

What was a child who was turning nine in the village of Love had to do?

A) Go to the Leader to receive a gift

B) Take on a mission to discover "The Big Secret"

C) Make a gift for the Leader

D) Be trained in the traditional arts of the village

How did the rosary beads help Helen?

A) They led her to the hidden lake

B) They showed her the way back to the village

C) They helped her solve a riddle

D) She discovered that they were magical and could talk

What was the big secret that Helen discovered?

A) A secret plan of the village

B) The discovery of her virtues and the wisdom to live them every day

C) A hidden treasure under the lake

D) An ancient magic potion

How did Helen react when she returned to the village?

A) She remained silent about her discovery

B) She shared the details of the secret with everyone.

C) She was sad and disappointed

D) She shared the wisdom and knowledge she had gained

Answer the following questions in complete sentences.

1. What was the significance of Helen's discovery of her virtues for her?

_____

_____

_____

_____

_____

2. What are your values for life and why?

_____

_____

_____

_____

_____

_____

_____

_____

_____

_____

_____

Put the events below in the correct order according to the text.

⇨ Helen solved the puzzle that led her to the hidden valley. _____

⇨ Helen returned to the village to share the wisdom she had gained. _____

⇨ Helen found a tall cypress tree and a manuscript underneath it. _____

⇨ Helen began her expedition with a map and a rosary. _____

⇨ Helen turned nine years old. _____

⇨ Helen realized the values she wanted to have in her life. _____

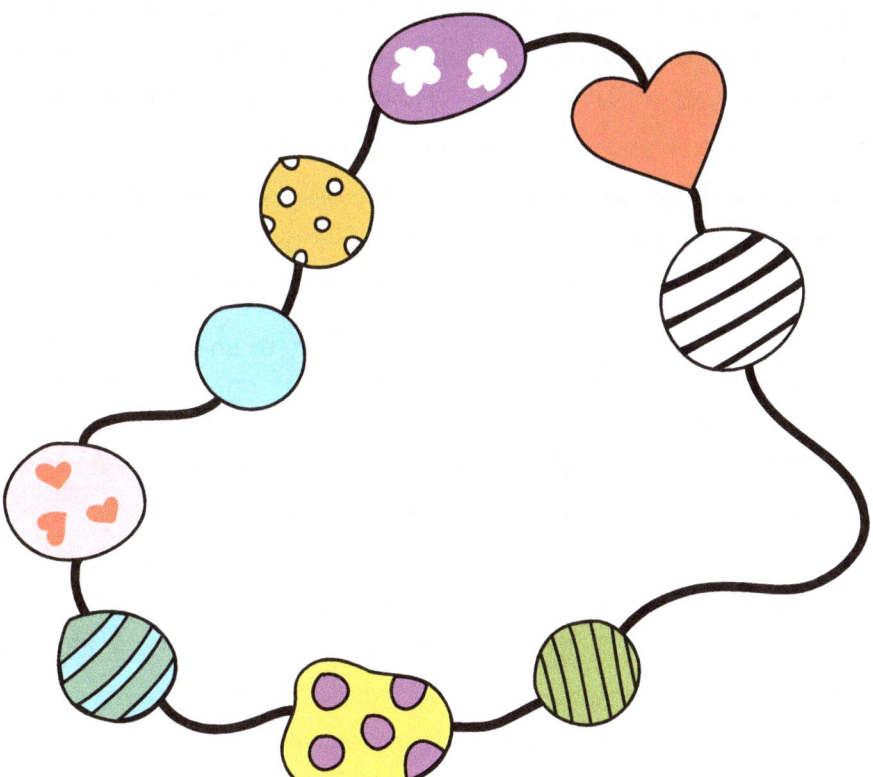

Read the texts carefully and solve the exercises.

The Camp

Summer was well underway and the Scout Troop decided to spend an exciting weekend at the "Starstone" camp. It was a camp in nature and all the children were looking forward to the day of departure.

All the children packed their backpacks very carefully. They packed everything they needed for the camping trip: sleeping bags, flashlights, and snacks for their daily adventures. The trip began with a song that echoed through the bus as it made its way through the trees and uphill.

Once they arrived, the kids pitched their tents near a lake with crystal clear waters. The groups were split up and each had their own mission. The scouts learned how to navigate with the help of the sun, how to safely start a fire, and how to build natural shelters.

When night fell the children gathered around the fire. They roasted various delicacies they had brought, and the scout leader told them stories about heroes who overcame difficulties and learned to respect and love nature.

The next day, the little scouts explored the forest trails, observed the animals, and collected leaves and stones to make constructions. They swam in the crystal clear lake waters and played group games.

The camp ended with a great treasure: the memory of an unforgettable adventure and the knowledge they gained. All the children returned home excited about the experiences they had and confident that nature is the greatest teacher and the perfect playground.

Mark the following sentences as True or False.

The camp "Starstone" was in the city. _____

The children learned how to make natural shelters. _____

The children arrived at the camp by train. _____

At night, the children sat around the fire and sang. _____

The camp experience helped the children to appreciate nature more. _____

Choose the correct answer.

Where were the children's tents placed?

A) In a meadow without trees

B) Near a lake with crystal clear waters

C) In a dark forest

D) At the edge of the village

What did the children do around the fire at night?

A) They told stories

B) They played hide and seek

C) They listened to music

D) They learned to dance

Which activity is NOT mentioned in the text that the children were doing?

A) Washing their clothes

B) Cooking by the fire.

C) Making natural shelters.

D) Collecting leaves and stones.

How did the children return from camp?

A) Disappointed

B) Smiling about their experience

C) Excited

D) Scared of the night

Answer the following questions in complete sentences.

1. What knowledge did the children gain from the camp?

_____

_____

_____

_____

_____

2. Why do you think the children felt that nature is "the perfect playground"?
Do you think so? Justify your answer.

_____

_____

_____

_____

_____

_____

_____

_____

_____

_____

_____

_____

_____

Put the events below in the correct order according to the text.

⇨ The camp ended with the memory of an unforgettable adventure.   _____

⇨ The children learned how to make natural shelters and how to
orient themselves.   _____

⇨ All the children returned home with a smile from the experience.   _____

⇨ The children arrived at camp and pitched their tents.   _____

⇨ They swam in the lake.   _____

Read the texts carefully and solve the exercises.

The new student

A new student, Linda, had come to Mark's class. Linda was a very introverted girl. She spoke very little and had a very low and soft voice. Some of her classmates began to tease her about it. Mark, who never missed the opportunity to make his classmates laugh, was usually the main perpetrator.

Linda never complained, nor had she ever complained to the teacher. She feared that the teasing would get worse if she spoke out. Usually after some teasing, she would lower her head and leave. Some days, she would go to the toilet and lock herself in until the bell rang, and others, she would wander past the teacher on call. That way, she felt safe that she was no longer in danger of getting teased by her classmates.

One afternoon, Mark was in his room doing homework when he heard his little sister burst into tears. He immediately ran to the living room where his sister was with his mom. "I don't want to go to school again," she cried, tears flowing in rivers. When Mark asked what had happened, his mom informed him that some kids were making fun of his sister at recess, which made her very sad. "I can't take it anymore. Please, Mom, let me stay home tomorrow," the girl said with teary eyes.

Seeing his sister in that state, Mark felt his stomach tied. He thought of Linda and all the times he and his classmates were amused by teasing and taunting her. Now, some other kids were doing the same to his sister and she was very sad, so much so that she didn't want to go back to school. It had never occurred to Mark that his teasing would upset Linda so much.

The next day, Mark went to school determined to fix what he had caused. Reluctantly but sincerely, he apologized to Linda for how he had treated her. She looked at him with both surprise and relief. After that, he never made fun of or teased Linda again, nor any other child. Even when other children teased, Mark didn't even laugh. He just changed the conversation with a serious tone.

Now, he knew how much pain a bad joke could cause. He promised that not only would he not tease anyone like that again, but he would try to stop it every time it happened. He understood that every action has consequences and that our words are powerful tools that can make the world a better or worse place—it's our choice.

Mark the following sentences as True or False.

Linda often complained to the teacher about her
classmates' teasing. _____

Mark never missed an opportunity to tease Linda. _____

Mark felt a knot in his stomach when he saw his sister crying
because she was being made fun of at school. _____

After the incident with his sister, Mark continued to tease Linda. _____

Mark promised to help stop the teasing at school. _____

Choose the correct answer.

How did Linda react to her classmates' teasing?

A) She told her teacher

B) She would lock herself in the bathroom or hang around the teacher

C) She would respond with teasing

D) She told her parents

What was one of the reasons the children made fun of Linda?

A) She didn't run fast

B) She didn't speak English

C) She had a low voice

D) She had a boyish voice

Why did Mark's sister not want to go to school?

A) Because she was sick

B) Because her friends were away

C) Because some children were making fun of her

D) Because she didn't like her courses

What did Mark feel when he realized that his sister had suffered the same thing as Linda?

A) Fear and guilt

B) Sadness and guilt

C) Joy and happiness

D) Anger and loneliness

How did Mark change after the incident with his sister?

A) He started making fun of other children

B) He became ashamed and changed school

C) He apologized to Linda and changed his behavior

D) He left school

Answer the questions in complete sentences.

1. How did Linda handle the teasing of her classmates? Would you do anything differently?

_____

_____

_____

_____

_____

_____

_____

_____

_____

_____

2. What made Mark change his attitude towards Linda and why?

_____
_____
_____
_____
_____
_____
_____
_____
_____
_____

Put the events below in the correct order according to the text.

⇨ Mark's sister didn't want to go to school because she was
   being made fun of.   _____

⇨ Mark felt guilty and promised himself never to make fun of
   others again.   _____

⇨ Linda was very sad and was hiding in the bathroom.   _____

⇨ Mark saw his sister crying and realized how much it hurts to
   be a victim of teasing.   _____

⇨ At first, Mark teased Linda with his other classmates.   _____

⇨ After his experience with his sister, Mark apologized to Linda. _____

Read the texts carefully and solve the exercises.

John's special Christmas

John and his family have been going on a trip to a European country every Christmas for the last seven years. It's something the whole family gets excited about because all the big cities are amazingly decorated for the holidays. Paris, London, Rome, and Vienna were among John's favorite Christmas destinations.

This year, however, things were somewhat different. A few days before Christmas, John's family decided to visit their grandfather in the village. Grandpa had recently been through a serious illness and they wanted to cheer him up and spend time with him. John was unhappy about this decision, but he couldn't help it, he was old enough to understand that Grandpa's health was a priority.

When they arrived, John helped his grandfather decorate the tree and the house. Grandpa taught him how to make traditional Christmas cookies, and they spent several hours in the kitchen, mixing, laughing, and telling stories from the first Christmas he and Grandma spent together.

On Christmas Eve, John helped his grandfather throw a small party for the neighbors. In the evening, the whole family sang traditional carols and exchanged small gifts. John felt a special bond with the village and its people. Life in the village was different, slower, and more peaceful, and Christmas was like something out of a fairy tale.

On Christmas night, as he gazed at the stars from the window, John realized that this Christmas was special because he spent many moments with his grandfather, learned a lot from him, and felt closer to his family and their traditions. So, he realized that the real value of Christmas lies not in the big, glamorous cities but in one's family and its bonds.

Mark the following sentences as True or False.

John visited his grandfather in the village a few days before Easter. _____

John and his grandfather made traditional Christmas cookies. _____

The village where Grandfather lived was called Snowflake. _____

On Christmas Eve, John stayed home and watched movies. _____

On Christmas night, John and his grandfather threw a party for

the neighbors. _____

Choose the correct answer.

What big city didn't John visit at Christmas?

A) Paris
B) London
C) Berlin
D) Vienna

What did John learn from his grandfather?

A) How to make toys
B) How to make traditional Christmas sweets
C) How to play chess
D) How to paint

Where was John's grandfather?

A) Near the sea
B) On a mountain
C) In a village
D) By a river

What was John's feeling about Christmas in the village?

A) Resentment

B) Excitement

C) Fear

D) Indifference

What did John do on Christmas Eve?

A) He played football

B) He helped throw a small party

C) He went shopping

D) He visited other relatives

How did John feel about this Christmas?

A) Disappointed

B) Happy

C) Anxious

D) Angry

Answer the questions in complete sentences.

1. How do you think John's experience in his grandfather's village changed his perception of Christmas?
Do you think the traditions and customs in the village affected the way he sees the holiday?

_____

_____

_____

_____

_____

_____

_____

2. How did you spend Christmas this year?

_____

_____

_____

_____

_____

_____

_____

_____

_____

_____

_____

_____

_____

_____

_____

_____

Put the events below in the correct order according to the text.

⇨ John learned how to make traditional cookies.   _____

⇨ John visited his grandfather in the village.   _____

⇨ John was not going to a big city for Christmas this year.   _____

⇨ John and his grandfather threw a party.   _____

⇨ John returned home after the holidays.   _____

Read the texts carefully and solve the exercises.

The advantages and the disadvantages of living in the city

The city is a place that many people choose to live, full of life and activities. However, like any place, the city has positive and negative aspects.

One of the city's advantages is that it offers plenty of work opportunities. From small businesses to large corporations, the options for work are countless. In addition, access to education and culture is greater in cities. There are many schools, universities, museums, and theatres that enrich everyday life. Finally, health services are more accessible, with many hospitals and clinics that offer advanced medical care.

On the other hand, there are many disadvantages to living in the city. Traffic can become unbearable due to the large number of cars. Also, cities often have high levels of air pollution. Noise is also a frequent source of discomfort, with sounds from traffic, construction, and other sources being part of everyday life.

In conclusion, city life is full of opportunities and challenges. Each individual must weigh the advantages and disadvantages to decide if the city is ideal for building their own life and finding happiness.

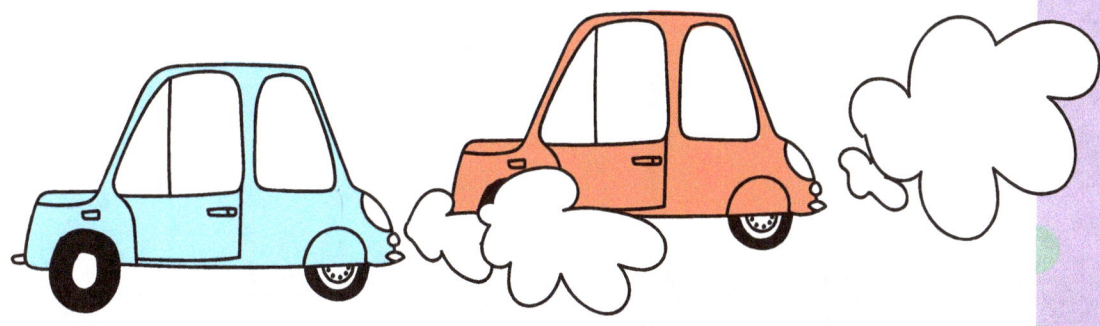

Mark the following sentences as True or False.

There are many opportunities for work in cities.　　　　　_____

Pollution is not a major problem in cities.　　　　　_____

Cities do not have many schools or universities.　　　　　_____

Noise in cities comes mainly from cars and construction.　　　　　_____

Traffic in cities is usually calm and easy.　　　　　_____

Choose the correct answer.

Which of the following is one of the positive aspects of the city?

A) High cost of living

B) Many job opportunities

C) Small variety of activities

D) Minimal health services

What is a major problem in cities?

A) Lack of housing

B) Pollution

C) Lack of schools

D) Lack of jobs

Which of the following is not a negative of the city?

A) Noise

B) Traffic

C) Easy access to education

D) Air pollution

Which of the following is a source of noise in cities?

A) Parks

B) Museums

C) Construction

D) Libraries

Where are a wide variety of hospitals and clinics located?

A) In rural areas

B) In cities

C) On islands

D) In mountainous areas

Answer the questions in complete sentences.

1. What are the main positive and negative aspects of city life?

_____

_____

_____

_____

_____

_____

_____

_____

_____

_____

2. Based on the text and your experience,
how do pollution and noise affect city life?

_____
_____
_____
_____
_____
_____
_____
_____
_____
_____

3. Where would you like to live? In the city or in the village, and why?

_____
_____
_____
_____
_____
_____
_____
_____
_____
_____
_____
_____
_____
_____

Read the texts carefully and solve the exercises.

The tree planting

On a bright and warm spring day, the school administration decided that all the 5th graders should dedicate the day to a special and important activity: planting trees in the schoolyard. Our teacher, Mr. Nick, who has a passion for nature, and Mrs. Penny, the other 5th-grade teacher, explained to us how important trees are for our life and the planet in general. With examples and vivid photos, they showed us how trees provide oxygen and shelter for animals while helping us reduce climate change consequences.

We all got excited, put on our gloves, and started working with enthusiasm. We divided into groups and each group took on a different activity: one group dug holes, another group placed the trees in the holes and a third group covered the holes with soil and watered the trees. Mr. Nick and Mrs. Penny proudly watched, encouraging and guiding us.

After a few weeks, the trees began to show the first signs of growth. Every day, we went during recess and watched the changes with excitement. Day by day, we noticed that a small animal world appeared around them: birds began building nests in the branches, while butterflies and bees visited their flowers. That was a real-life lesson as we realized that by planting trees we were not only making our school more beautiful but also contributing to the improvement of the whole ecosystem and a better future for all of us. Even the smallest act, like planting a tree, could make a big difference to our planet.

Mark the following sentences as True or False.

The 5th-grade children planted trees in the fall. _____

Mr. Nick and Mrs. Mary teach the 5th grade. _____

The trees started to grow the following year. _____

After planting, the children observed birds building nests. _____

Planting trees improves the whole ecosystem. _____

Choose the correct answer.

The teachers explained that the trees:

A) Should be watered daily

B) Provide oxygen and shelter for animals.

C) Should be planted in everyone's home

D) Need to be pruned to grow stronger

How did the children feel when planting the trees?

A) Bored

B) Excited

C) Scared

D) Indifferent

Which of the following did the children not do during the tree planting?

A) They pruned the trees

B) Watered the trees

C) They dug holes

D) They filled the holes with soil

What did the children learn from this experience?

A) To dig holes

B) The value of trees in the ecosystem

C) To water plants

D) To rune trees

Answer the questions in complete sentences.

1. Based on the text and your own experiences,
why do you think it is crucial to plant trees in our cities?

_____

_____

_____

_____

_____

_____

_____

_____

_____

_____

_____

_____

_____

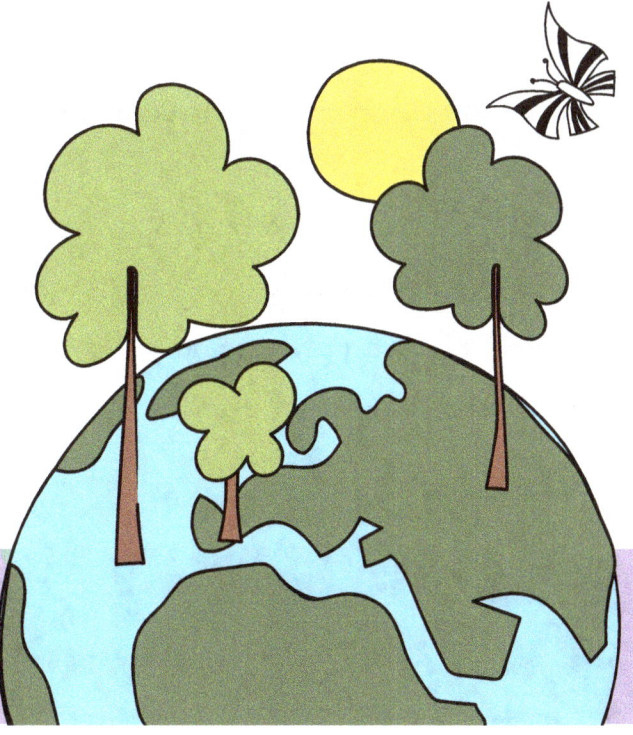

2. What other measures do you think could help protect the environment?

_____

_____

_____

_____

_____

_____

_____

_____

_____

_____

_____

_____

_____

_____

_____

_____

Put the events below in the correct order according to the text.

⇨ The trees began to grow, and the birds began to build nests
  on their branches.   _____

⇨ Mr. Nick and Mrs. Penny explained the importance of trees in nature.   _____

⇨ The children put on their gloves and started planting the trees.   _____

⇨ The 5th-grade teachers decided to plant trees in the schoolyard.   _____

⇨ The children realized the real value of tree planting.   _____

Read the texts carefully and solve the exercises.

The children's online life

Nowadays, technology has become an integral part of our daily lives. This is especially true for children since they come into contact with various electronic devices from a very young age. From smartphones and tablets to computers and game consoles, technology offers children new ways to learn, have fun, and communicate. But at the same time, it also brings challenges that need to be addressed wisely.

Education through technology can be very rewarding. Children have access to a vast world of information and can explore various interesting topics. Many educational apps help to deepen knowledge through games and activities that are both fun and educational.

On the other hand, online life can also have negative aspects. Excessive exposure in front of a screen can have physical health effects, such as resulting in vision problems or obesity. In addition, online safety is an important issue. Children need to learn how to protect their personal data and how to recognize potentially dangerous situations.

Another factor is social interaction. While social networks and communication applications allow children to keep in touch with friends and family, there is a risk that they may lose contact with the real world. In addition, cyberbullying has become a serious threat, as the anonymity of the internet encourages some to behave irresponsibly or be hostile.

Children must learn how to balance their online with their real lives. Parents and teachers need to be aware of and discuss with children the challenges and opportunities that technology offers. Through guidance and appropriate education, children can reap the benefits of technology while maintaining a healthy balance in their lives.

Mark the following sentences as True or False.

Technology provides children only with positive experiences and opportunities. _____

Educational apps help children learn through fun games and activities. _____

Excessive use of electronic devices has no effect on children's physical health. _____

Online bullying is not a significant problem for children online. _____

Parents and teachers should discuss the challenges and opportunities of technology with children. _____

Children need to learn how to protect their personal data online. _____

Choose the correct answer.

What is one of the effects of excessive use of screens?

A) Vision problems
B) Improved memory
C) Increased physical activity
D) None of the above

How does technology help in the education of children?

A) Limits access to information
B) Provides access to a rich world of information
C) Reduces interest in learning
D) None of the above

Which of the following is not a problem associated with technology?

A) Obesity
B) Cyberbullying
C) Ease of communication
D) Loss of privacy

Why is it important for children to learn how to balance their online lives?

A) To increase the use of technology

B) To maintain a healthy balance in their lives

C) To avoid physical exercise

D) To become technology experts

Which of the following is a way to protect yourself online?

A) Sharing personal information

B) Not identifying dangerous situations

C) Protection of personal data

D) Avoiding communication with friends

What is the role of parents and teachers in children's technological education?

A) To prevent the use of technology

B) To be informed and discuss challenges and opportunities

C) To ignore technological changes

D) To focus only on the negative aspects

Answer the questions in complete sentences.

1. What are the positive and negative aspects of children's online life?

_____

_____

_____

_____

_____

_____

_____

_____

_____

2. What are the positive and negative aspects of your own online life?

_____

_____

_____

_____

_____

_____

_____

_____

_____

_____

_____

3. Over time, do you think the positive aspects of children's use of technology outweigh the negative or vice versa?

_____

_____

_____

_____

_____

_____

_____

_____

_____

_____

_____

_____

The value of volunteering

Imagine a world where everyone helps everyone. A world full of cooperation, empathy, and solidarity. That's the model world that volunteering aims to create. Volunteering is giving without expecting a reward. It's the opportunity to help others simply to feel better, not because you must. It's a way to build a better future.

Volunteering is very important these days. Through volunteering you can help people who really need it. This can be helping the elderly, participating in environmental care projects, or supporting social events. Every effort counts and makes a difference.

In addition, volunteering helps a person to develop new skills. While contributing to a good cause, they also learn how to work with others, solve problems, organize events, and much more depending on the type of volunteering they do. The volunteer develops skills that are important for the rest of their lives.

Volunteering even helps to meet new people. Meeting other volunteers and people from different places and cultures. That means new friendships and new experiences. Several volunteer actions take place abroad, and they are valuable life lessons because you learn about other people's lives and share your own.

In addition, volunteering gives you a feeling of fulfillment and satisfaction. When you see the positive impact of your actions on the lives of others or the community, it gives you a sense of moral satisfaction. It's a feeling that no salary can give you, no matter how high.

Wondering how you can become a volunteer? First, start at your school. Discuss with your school administration what needs there are and whether it's possible to fulfill any. Maybe it's cleaning a part of the school or planting trees. Then, you can continue with the community you live in. Find out about local organizations that need help. You can also talk to your teachers or parents to find ways to help. Every little contribution is important.

Volunteering is a way to open the door to helping each other and the community. It's an opportunity to show sensitivity, care, and love for others. When we help, we make the world a little brighter and more hopeful for all of us.

Mark the following sentences as True or False.

Volunteering is only about helping the elderly. _____

Through volunteering, you can learn new skills, such as cooperation. _____

Volunteering offers you a good salary. _____

Volunteering can help in making new friendships and getting to
know different cultures. _____

To become a volunteer you must always belong to a specific
organization. _____

Choose the correct answer.

What is one of the benefits of volunteering?

A) Earning money

B) Learning new skills

C) Providing services

D) Opportunity to travel

What is not volunteering?

A) Cleaning up the local community

B) Helping the elderly

C) Giving gifts to children in need

D) Planting school trees

How can you volunteer?

A) By paying a membership fee

B) Via the internet

C) By learning about local organizations and talking to teachers or parents

D) By getting a special diploma

What is the feeling that volunteering gives you?

A) Jealousy

B) Indifference

C) Satisfaction

D) Tiredness

What is one reason that makes volunteering important?

A) It helps promote personal interests

B) It provides material goods

C) It helps people in need

D) It secures job opportunities

Answer the questions in complete sentences.

1. Describe an experience or activity you would like to volunteer for and why.

_____

_____

_____

_____

_____

_____

_____

_____

_____

_____

_____

2. Think of a skill you would like to develop through volunteering.
How would this skill help you in your daily life?

_____
_____
_____
_____
_____
_____
_____
_____
_____
_____
_____

3. How do you think volunteering can help improve the local community
where you live?

_____
_____
_____
_____
_____
_____
_____
_____
_____
_____
_____
_____

4. Think of a time when you felt satisfied helping someone else.
Describe the moment and how it made you feel.

_____

_____

_____

_____

_____

_____

_____

_____

_____

_____

_____

_____

_____

_____

_____

_____

_____

_____

_____

_____

_____

_____

_____

_____